Prayer Prescriptions For Nurse Healers

Kate Loving Shenk RN BSN

Copyright@2012

Kate Loving Shenk RN/BSN

All rights reserved.

No part of this publication may be reproduced, distributed or transmitted in any form or by any means, including photocopying, recording or other electronic or mechanical methods, without the prior permission of the author, except in the case of brief quotations embodied in critical reviews and certain noncommercial uses permitted by copyright law.

Contents

DEDICATION PAGE
viii

A Note To My Readers
ix

Disclaimer
xi

How To Connect With Kate Loving Shenk
xii

PART ONE: SLEEP WORKING WITHIN THE PATRIARCHAL MEDICAL SYSTEM
xiv

CHAPTER ONE: WORK PREPARATION AND NURSING EDUCATION
xvi

CHAPTER TWO: THE NURSE/DOCTOR RELATIONSHIP
xxi

CHAPTER THREE: THE NURSE-PATIENT RELATIONSHIP
xxviii

CHAPTER FOUR: NURSES EAT THEIR YOUNG
xxxiii

CHAPTER FIVE: MODELS AND MENTORS
xxxvi

CHAPTER SIX: NURSE PRACTITIONER AUTONOMY
xl

CHAPTER SEVEN: THE MEDICAL GESTAPO
xlix

CHAPTER EIGHT: BURN OUT
lv

CHAPTER NINE: TIME CLOCK TYRANNY
lix

PART TWO: WAKING UP IN THE PATRIARCHAL MEDICAL SYSTEM
lxii

CHAPTER TEN: MUSSOLINIAN LEADERSHIP
lxiii

CHAPTER ELEVEN: POVERTY MEDICINE
lxvi

CHAPTER TWELVE: WELFARE TO WORK
lxix

CHAPTER THIRTEEN: INSPIRED LIVING VERSUS LOSS OF VISION
lxxiii

CHAPTER FOURTEEN: DAILY WORK
lxxvii

CHAPTER FIFTEEN: TRANSFORMING THE BATTLEGROUND
lxxx

CHAPTER SIXTEEN: MERGING ALLOPATHIC AND COMPLEMENTARY MEDICINE
lxxxiii

CHAPTER SEVENTEEN: PATHOLOGICAL OPTIMISM
lxxxviii

CHAPTER EIGHTEEN: ADVOCACY
xcii

CHAPTER NINETEEN: WORK PLACE DIVERSITY
xcvi

CHAPTER TWENTY: NATIONAL HEALTH INSURANCE IN AMERICA
civ

CHAPTER TWENTY-ONE: FLOW AND RESILIENCE AND ECSTATIC STATES OF MIND
cxv

CHAPTER TWENTY-TWO: THE ART AND SCIENCE AND MEDICINE
cxx

CHAPTER TWENTY-THREE: MYSTICS IN THE WORKPLACE
cxxvii

PART THREE: STAYING AWAKE: CREATING COMPASSION
cxxxii

CHAPTER TWENTY-FOUR: FROM BASEMENT TO BOUNDARY
cxxxii

CHAPTER TWENTY-FIVE: DOING TIME ON PLANET EARTH
cxxxvi

CHAPTER TWENTY-SIX: THE ANGELS ARE WITH US

cxxxviii

CHAPTER TWENTY-SEVEN: ANGELS OF MERCY
cxl

CHAPTER TWENTY-EIGHT: THE END OF HUMAN DOMINION
cxlii

CHAPTER TWENTY-NINE: RELINGUISHING THE EGO
cxlvii

CHAPTER THIRTY: TEARS AND HEALING
cl

CHAPTER THIRTY-ONE: LISTENING
clii

CHAPTER THIRTY-TWO: PRACTICING FORGIVENESS
cliv

CHAPTER THIRTY-THREE: BALANCE AND PROTECTION
clvi

CHAPTER THIRTY-FOUR: AGEISM
clviii

CHAPTER THIRTY-FIVE: SUFFERING

clx

CHAPTER THIRTY-SIX: COMPASSION
clxii

CHAPTER THIRTY-SEVEN: ATTRACTION/AVERSION
clxiv

CHAPTER THIRTY-EIGHT: TRANSFORMATION OF THE SELF
clxvi

CHAPTER THIRTY-NINE: TRANSFORMING THE MEDICAL SYSTEM
clxviii

CHAPTER FORTY: HEALING AND THE NATURAL WORLD
clxix

CHAPTER FORTY-ONE: LIFE IS BUT A DREAM
clxxii

CHAPTER FORTY-TWO: THE NEW YEARS BABY
clxxiv

Connect With Kate
clxxviii

Bibliography
clxxx

Dedication Page

This book is dedicated to all nursing students and future students of the world who in the great spirit of Florence Nightingale, want to hold up the candle and light the pathway for those so called to follow, in the hope that health care can be humanized and stripped of all barriers to compassion in service and in care.

Om Peace Amen

A Note To My Readers

I have been a nurse for 28 years. One of the things we must ask our patients is if they have a spiritual or religious practice that gives them comfort.

More often than not, a patient will simply say, "I pray."

Naturally, I understand exactly what they mean. No further explanation is necessary.

Prayer puts people on a level playing field. As more and more people admit to their practice of prayer, we can learn to throw our prayers into a hat, and pass the good will around.

Prayer is love. Prayer heals. It clears your heart, so that only the good is drawn to you forever.

Prayer Prescriptions For Nurse Healers is the first in a series of Prayer Prescription books.

This book is my prayer prescription for nurses everywhere.

May you be happy. May you be well. May you find peace of mind.

These prayer prescriptions are a series of

stories about my life as a nurse. Some would call it a Nurse Memoir, but I am calling it a Nurse's Prayer Prescription.

The next book in the prayer prescription series, is called: *Prayer Prescriptions: Spiritual Remedies For Long Lasting Health*. After that one, *Prayer Prescriptions For Vagina Sisterhood, A Manifesto For Nurses*.

Read this book, and be guided to your own Prayer Prescription. Have faith in its ability to heal. Love awaits all who embrace prayer prescriptions into their lives. And even those who don't.

Disclaimer

I have tried to recreate events, locales and conversations from my memories of them. In order to maintain their anonymity in some instances I have changed the names of individuals and places, I may have changed some identifying characteristics and details such as physical properties, occupations and places of residence.

This book is not intended as a substitute for the medical advice of physicians. The reader should regularly consult a physician in matters relating to his/her health and particularly with respect to any symptoms that may require diagnosis or medical attention.

How To Connect With Kate Loving Shenk RN/BSN

SUBSCRIBE AND RECEIVE A FREE REPORT: _22 Keys To Self Healing_, plus Prayer Prescriptions Delivered to your email nearly every day!

http://katelovingshenk.com

Facebook Fan Pages: Kate's Radio Show Fan Page

https://www.facebook.com/KateLovingCreativeWisdom

Kate's Author Page: https://www.facebook.com/kate2233

Kate's Blue Heron Farm Spiritual Retreat Center Fan Page On Facebook:

https://www.facebook.com/BlueHeronFarmRetreat

Kate's Prayer Prescription For Nurse Healer Fan Page On Face Book: https://www.facebook.com/PrayerPrescriptionsForNurseHealers?ref=hl

Twitter: https://twitter.com/kateloving

Linked In:
http://www.linkedin.com/in/katelovingshenk22

PRAYER PRESCRIPTIONS FOR NURSE HEALERS is the first in a series. The next book is called: *PRAYER PRESCRIPTIONS: SPIRITUAL REMEDIES FOR LONG LASTING HEALTH.* I plan to write *PRAYER PRESCRIPTIONS FOR AGING GRACEFULLY*, *PRAYER PRESCRIPTIONS FOR THE LOVE OF OUR ANIMAL COMPANIONS*, *PRAYER PRESCRIPTIONS FOR VAGINA SISTERHOOD, A NURSING MANIFESTO*

PART ONE: Sleep Working Within the Patriarchal Medical System

I am walking through the long corridors of the hospital where I work. The nurses dispense medicines and chart on the medical record. Sick patients walk the hallways for exercise. Somber pictures of male doctors who have retired in the many years since the hospital's beginnings line the elevator foyers. I do not see one picture of a woman, doctor or nurse.

These pictures represent the patriarchal system, sending a message: not of male domination, but the domination of a life force that is solemn and unyielding. This tyrannical world view is what people face going to work every day in the business, education and medical world, and in the factory. People spend over one half of their lives on the job, feeling unsupported and alienated.

As my friend Steve said the other night, while reminiscing about one of his many jobs in the world: "No one laughed in that factory, not even a smile."

Everyone at the table nodded in recognition, with nothing to add to the statement. We were safe in our kitchen, with Mukunda the dog playing ball with any willing person. The steady light of the night stars were present from every window. The battle ground of the patriarchy would begin again Monday, at 8:00 a.m.

Chapter One: Work Preparation and Nursing Education

My mother always wanted me to be a nurse. Why not a doctor, a writer, a violinist? For that matter, why not a lion trainer, a tight rope walker or zookeeper? She said she saw it in my Astrological Chart, all the planetary configurations aligned to equal nurse, spelled by stars across the night sky.

I've been a Nurse Practitioner since 1987 and a registered nurse since 1984- and have been a clinical nurse mentor to many students since that time. I've taught them practical skills and have made sure they follow protocols of good practice.

Yet what I really want them to learn is difficult to teach; and that is, how to approach patients non - judgmentally, how to look upon the patient's situation with compassion, no matter how dire the circumstances or how responsible the person is for her predicament. I want my students to learn the great value of dealing exclusively with people, to learn to read them and to know them.

One of the first perils along this pathway is the slippery task of completing nursing school education.

After I get to know each of my students, she usually reveals the crisis that shattered her soul in nursing school. She tells how she moved on in life, a wounded but wiser person.

I remember my first sight when I entered the Obstetrical/Gynecological Nurse Practitioner classroom for the first time where nearly sixteen of us spent each learning session together for the next three months: thirty-two stacks of books, from floor to ceiling, two stacks apiece of required reading.

We lived in a high rise complex in center city Philadelphia, just a few blocks from where Jeffrey Dommer was cannibalizing young women. We came to know this later. Four of us lived on the twentieth floor, two women to a room, overlooking a tree line and a Philadelphia boulevard down below.

I shared a double bed with a perfect stranger, whose name was Erin. She had blue eyes, the color of the deepest well. We talked and smoked cigarettes. We spoke of our fear of failing grades, of our childhood, of the loneliness of big city noises and black night skies, illuminated by street lights and the grey hue of car and truck pollution.

The Nurse Practitioner course moved along at a rapid speed that caused great discomfort among my fellow students. Traditionally, the transition from the role of Registered Nurse to Nurse Practitioner is one at best that churns the intestines with unease.

My one roommate, Ursula, the smartest woman in the class, was always running to the bathroom before a test, expelling all of her anxiety into the toilet. We worried that if the smartest one among us was so nervous, what were we to do? We all had our distinctive way to express our worry about getting through, surviving and "passing" the program.

One night Erin came home, waving a pair of white pants. She stood on the balcony and threw the white pants into the wind, and all four of us watched as the pants make a flapping sound all the way to the street below.

She turned to us and explained that the pants represented her mother, that now her mother will be liberated, and so will she. At first, she calmly explained this, then she became more and more excited by the insights elicited by this event.

I knew that Erin was not excelling in the clinical setting, although she was doing well in the didactic arena. Everyday, we were going into the hospital or clinic, mostly in inner city Philadelphia, where we received a crash course in human disease, sadness and desperation.

The women we cared for were criminals or street people or both, sometimes taken directly from the prison to the clinic in hand cuffs, to receive medical intervention for vaginal bleeding, sexually transmitted infections, HIV related illness or a combination of all of these things, and more.

After the pants touched down, we retired to our room. Erin could not sleep, and her reasoning ability went the way of the white pants, becoming tattered by the rolling traffic of incessant thought.

I moved back to my home sixty miles away, and became a commuter, so that I could concentrate on the huge amount of school work I needed to complete, in order to pass. Erin soon left the program.

As we spent those many nights talking before her breakdown, a slow dawning realization jolted my mind: Erin reminded me of my first husband, with her fathomless deep blue eyes, with her far away looks, in just the way she explained certain phenomenon. I never told her this, which is a good thing. I've often wondered who I reminded her of, and what it means to be struck by a person's likeness in totally unfamiliar circumstances.

I never did read all of those books, but learned to balance a speculum on my forehead, and play spoons with a jug band on the busy city corner down the street.

Chapter Two: The Nurse/Doctor Relationship

I used to work at a large teaching hospital. We imparted our expertise to the student doctors in the bowels of the hospital basement where steam pipes and heating systems sent power throughout the health system. The neighboring morgue quietly collected those who had died.

The hush of the basement hallway led to a nondescript door, where inside, resident training took place, and where the indigent were sent to receive medical care.

This is where we spent most of our days, without natural light, without a window, with the glare of fluorescence beaming light on the business of ringing phones and constant talk, on the sadness and joy of the patients who came and went.

I was in the middle of taking a complex history from a patient who had multiple problems. She was homeless. She was a heroin addict. Her children had been placed in foster homes, all with different foster parents.

She had pain in her lower abdomen with erratic menstrual cycles. She may be pregnant again. If this was a pregnancy in her tubes, she could die.

I realized I would have to go over this story with the chief Obstetrical/Gynecological resident. He was weeks away from joining the practice of his dreams. His four year residency was almost over.

I explained to him the patient's predicament, her medical problems, the differential diagnosis, and then my plan. I sensed impatience on his part as he shuffled papers, refused to give eye contact, shifted his weight in the chair where he sat.

I experienced this with him and his contemporaries every day of my working life there, and I thought -when will medical schools start teaching these doctors how to relate to their patients?

Where are all the saints when we need them?

I didn't like my students to see this kind of all too frequent attitude of the resident doctors. Many times, I would shield them from it, had them continue to listen to a patient, to see what insights they could share with me about her life and her health.

But nursing education addresses the

dichotomy of the nurse/doctor relationship in the classroom all the time. This is something we all know about. We know the history of it. Nurses are no longer physician handmaidens, but we suspect the doctors would like us to be.

I remember many other chief residents who spent three years being beaten and trodden upon by other chief residents, attending physicians and yes, probably even nurses. By the time they assume the fourth year chief resident position of responsibility for each patient that comes for care, they are afflicted, mean and ready to be cruel to anyone they can as a payback.

Egocentricity has been hammered into the very core of their beings. They are unlikely to ever give it up in this life time.

I perceived an especially vicious attitude towards the nurses who had their own case load of Obstetric patients. These nurses did home visits and saw the patients individually when they come to our facility for prenatal care.

They taught, involved themselves in family dynamics and developed relationships that patients never forgot.

One of my colleagues made her insights about various patients known routinely to the chief resident. This should have been welcomed knowledge to him. A collaborative plan could have been created to make the nurse's expert observations apart of the broad plan of care.

But my friend was routinely mocked by this upper level resident. One time, he screamed at her in front of patients and staff about a decision she made.

My friend recently left the nursing profession to become a minister.

I, too, had been the sadistic target of these doctors. I remember a huge woman, Dr. O., who had grown more hateful with each passing year of her residency. She began a rampage of terror the first week as chief resident, year four of her residency. I over heard her on the phone making loud demands to the medical records and pharmacy staff, to the nurse manager and above all, to lower level residents.

I began a new schedule one afternoon a week without any residents or attending physicians in the clinic. This meant that I saw patients in a peaceful setting. If I had a question, I could make a call and get the answer. I was told that Dr. O. asked around to other nurses and secretaries about my credentialing. I heard her snicker to another doctor about my new afternoon clinic as if I was incapable of doing the job I have done for the past fifteen years.

One of the new first year residents and I found ourselves in the microscope room together. I asked her how she was doing. She said, "I've learned more than I've ever learned in so short a period. But I also have never been so abused." There was a pause. Of course I knew where the shaft was coming from.

She went on. "My birthday was the other day. I'd been complaining to my husband and (seven year old) daughter about these constant assaults on my spirit. My daughter came to the clinic, marched right up to Dr. O. and said,

"Have you been nice to my mommy today? It is her birthday."

Dr. O. glared at the new resident and her eyes narrowed. "What have you been telling her?" And then she was called away to answer a call.

The new resident could have said, "Oh, I was just using you as an example of how not to treat other people."

One of my favorite obnoxious fourth year chief

residents was once a nurse, now Doctor. She seemed to hate nurses more than any of the other doctors, if that is possible. She singled out mistakes made by anyone of the nursing staff and would point out the stupidity of the person in front of patients and their families. It didn't matter who was around.

She was also particular about exactly how she wanted everything to be set up in an exam room. She expected a nurse to wait on her, giving her the necessary tool and ordered her around in front of the patient if the task was not done just so.

She ate greasy hamburgers and french fries for lunch every day. I never saw her eat one single vegetable or piece of fruit.

She went into a private practice in the area and one of our freshly hired nurses was employed to work for her.

I hear she is no longer a practicing nurse.

I ascended the steps leading out of the basement at the end of the day. The sun was setting. I squinted like a mole who had been unearthed. I walked my student to her car.

"How do you feel about the clinic?" I asked.

"It definitely is a learning experience," was her comment. "Is that good or bad?" I ask.

"I'm not sure. I'll have to think about it."

And many spirited discussions resulted in the ensuing days about the nursing profession, health care in general and the future of medicine in America.

And these students still want to be Nurse Practitioners. They hoped that someday, doctors and nurses can develop equal relationships based on mutual respect. And that most of all, nurses are finally revered for the contributions they make.

It is time to realize that health care will collapse if there are no more nurses.

Chapter Three: The Nurse-Patient Relationship

The beauty about the profession of nursing is that we can practice in different settings and specialties over the course of our working lives. We live multi-dimensional lives, many lives within the course of one life, with rebirths and awakenings, all in the span of 25-40 years.

Original research is what I was after as I was writing this book. Nurse Practitioner work kept me busy with in the confines of an office and clinic environment.

Yet the real battleground of our profession lies in the hospital doing bedside nursing, ministering to the cares and concerns of patients who are more than likely terrified of being in the hands of doctors and nurses, many for the first time.

In 2003, I signed up for a labor and delivery nursing position, to observe the world of nursing from an entirely different perspective. The specialty was infinitely more complex than I wanted to admit, at first. The sheer amount of work involved with every aspect of the process had to be mastered.

As a newly hired person, the doctors and nurse

midwives were not happy to be working with someone who was not in total command of the situation. But who ever is? Yet over time, we all became more comfortable with one another.

The nurse at the bedside is the person who sees first hand the state of mind, the physical well being or physical deterioration of the patient over many hours. This is an opportunity to build a relationship of trust and a healing atmosphere around the bedside. A sacred protection develops and "time" no longer exists, in any linear framework.

An attitude of reverence settles over my psyche the moment my first step reaches the hospital entrance. I feel a sense of peace, of higher purpose as I set out to meet the unknown. A feeling of helper, of servant, of humility overtakes my general attitude.

Yet before I actually arrive to the institution, I may feel anxious or overburdened by the critical challenges ahead. But this uneasiness dissipates. I do meditate before each work session: a highly recommended act for achieving peace of mind and serenity.

Out of this arises a love that supersedes understanding. The great feeling of service overtakes everything. It feels like other forces are at work to make this happen, especially the angels. I remember with purpose to call upon the angels on the twenty minute drive to the hospital. And they always respond. This I know without doubt.

Emergency situations arise routinely in the Labor and Delivery arena.. As a Nurse Practitioner for sixteen years, I did not see many emergencies and when they occurred, we called for help. The patient was immediately transferred out of the area after CPR was administered, when needed.

I worked the full moon, recently. One of our patients that evening had a seizure originating from a pregnancy related complication. Another patient was rushed to the operating room after her uterus ruptured.

Several patients arrived and delivered their babies quickly within the quarter hour, and we all helped one another with tasks that needed to be done, meanwhile reassuring patients and families that everything was being done to assure a safe and healthy outcome.

The stronger and more loving the bond between a nurse and her patient, the less likely a lawsuit will arise. Yet obstetrics is at the center of malpractice litigation in America today. The specialty is driven by the latest lawsuit and how to avoid another one.

Fear of the courts and of the professional ruin that results haunts our practice like a stubborn, unyielding ghost.

A word about nursing codependency: We are the greatest co-dependents in the universe. Yet a distinct line exists between the altruistic urge to care for and meet our patients needs with generosity, and the codependents need to help, arising from a lack of self-love or self-nurturing.

Codependency breeds a tendency to resent the needs of others, but to continue to perform acts of service in a mood of resentment that often cannot be hidden by a tone of voice that sounds rushed, or even hostile.

And this hostility is the tip-off that the patient is in the way or is a bother-and the patient knows it.

The love I am referring to that a nurse has for her patient is devoid entirely of codependency. It is a feeling that originates from the magnetic pull of love for the Beloved or the God of your understanding-an urge that speaks to the calling that all good nurses have regarding their profession.

The calling that may take a lifetime to understand.

Chapter Four: Nurses Eat Their Young

We were discussing the nurse calling the other evening, about ten P. M., three hours into my twelve hour shift; the labor and delivery nursing job that has helped me understand the mind of registered nurses, in this one place but as expressed in hospitals all over the planet.

My colleagues were at least twenty-five years younger than myself, all of them claiming to be there for the same reason-to serve, to help and to honor their patients.

Victoria, one of the nurses said, "Why do nurses eat their young? Why are they so mean to the new graduates or to the newly hired women?"

And every women there proceeded to tell a story of mistreatment in the first days and weeks of the new job on the Labor and Delivery unit.

"Is this because we are working with other women? Women are notorious for selling each other down the river," I said.

And the nurse whose mind set is strict or patronizing need not be "old." She may be just several years out of school. But the old codependency issue comes to mind. The nurse who snaps at the freshly hired graduate often is in a mind set of perfection, thinking she is the only one who can do the job and would never think to ask for help.

These qualities of the need to control with passive/aggressive undertones are what meet most of us as we work with other nurses.

One beautiful and caring young women described a scenario of being screamed at when she skipped a step in setting up an epidural pump. This negativity washed over her like a tsunami and she had to go home immediately and cry for the rest of the day.

She thought about applying for other work, leaving nursing altogether. Many of us develop a hardened exterior over time so that the negative vibrations no longer seemingly have an effect. But they always do, especially among the more sensitive or vulnerable in our midst.

A fearless approach to inner exploration, healthy self-examination and a willingness to change and to seek inner peace is needed among women in our profession.

Nurse, Heal Thyself-and Physician, too.

The inner reservoirs for self-healing are like the deepest well–endless and fathomless.

Chapter Five: Models and Mentors

I always want to tell my student to pick out a heroic doctor or nurse-one that my student can totally relate to and wants to be like in every way- and copy the heroic model until the student feels like she is that person. She can walk, talk and sing like her hero until suddenly, one day, she has a practice with a following.

This creative process is like being an actor or actress, when only after all the lines are memorized can the character come alive in the psyche. The danger lies in becoming lost in the process, not knowing where the play acting ends and the newly found self begins.

But I say: you can't possibly fail if you really want to become a better person, and a better health care provider, as a result.

My all time revered mentor has retired after forty years of service. I worked with him every day for nine years, and he was responsible for hiring me as a Nurse Practitioner in the first place.

His portrait has joined the groups of smile-less paintings of male doctors throughout the hospital. But his portrait is different, and thus in obvious contrast, people will stop and look.

His is not a somber face. Instead, his mouth forms a Mona Lisa smile as he stands at a black board with his own simulated hand writing detailing a child's medical history in a list beside him on the board, a piece of chalk held in his right hand, about to write another point in the patients history.

He is, and always will be, the Pediatric Guru.

When he did come back to the clinic, to fill in for a vacationing doctor, we'd all rejoice. The aura of the clinic was raised a million fold. When he left, the energy fields collapsed.

It was a major social event when he came back. Patients and staff always wanted to know what he was doing. He listened intently to their recent stories concerning family and friends. He interjected advice that fit. I remember when our dear Raphael, now twenty-two years of age, came in after his girl friend had a pregnancy loss and he was trying to make sense of it. The good doctor listened.

He told Raphael that he had seen him live through the loss of his mother, and a cardiac valve replacement after a bout of rheumatic fever. He gave Raphael the confidence to see his way through the crisis because of their twenty-two year bond and comradery.

Many times, a patient had something to say and would not say it. There was an unexpressed pain in the eye, an unconscious tense clasp of hands, a silence born of constant sadness. I approached the problem from several perspectives but couldn't elicit the real truth of what was bothering the person.

Finally, after thirty minutes of asking, consoling and even silence, I called in the Pediatric Guru.

He strolled into the room, over to the baby or child, talked to the child, picked up the baby. The baby pulled his white beard and he laughed. He took out a well worn alligator finger puppet and delighted the child or children with a hide-and-go seek game, or a tweak to the nose for a round of giggles.

The child took the alligator puppet, and we settled down to speak with the parent. Often, the child would go out to play with a nurse in the playroom. Then the father or mother revealed a deepest fear, a most unsettling anxiety. This was done in the time it takes the night heron to soundlessly wing several miles to bullfrog music on a midsummer's evening.

Mukunda the dog loves the Pediatric Guru. He patiently waits in the car while we all go dancing or to restaurants to eat and talk or to Saint Patrick's Day celebrations where we play Fisherman's Blues and Fiddler's Green.

Sometimes, he waits while we dance with feet moving fast to disco beats and balls of crystal lights rotating like globes with refracting strobes pulsing the eye at various angles. Then, at the end of it all, we take Pediatric Guru to see Mukunda, who barks and leaps merrily around this Irish leprechaun.

My mentor is now my friend–the greatest gift of all.

Chapter Six: Nurse Practitioner Autonomy

Nurse Practitioner practice was regulated by both the Board of Medicine and the Board of Nursing in the state of Pennsylvania until very recently. Most states only require regulation by the nursing board, which is the way we wanted it in Pennsylvania. But the fight to achieve this spanned a twenty year period.

The compromise was to give Nurse Practitioners prescriptive authority and to keep the dual regulation. Nurse Practitioners in almost every state already had prescriptive authority.

So we are in the dark ages here in Pennsylvania. But prescriptive authority did finally pass in Pennsylvania, one of the last states to conform to this ruling. And the Board of Medicine no longer regulates Nurse Practitioner practice.

My specialty and certification is Women's Health. I also practiced fifteen years as a Pediatric Nurse Practitioner with mentors such as the pediatric guru. The knowledge gleaned from the expertise of the great doctor and others is not easily passed on in the context of a regimented educational course of study.

Prescriptive privilege legislation was accompanied by a regulatory crackdown that over the course of several years, forced me to abandon my entire Nurse Practitioner practice. So I ask myself and my general audience: does prescriptive authority expand or narrow the role of Nurse Practitioner? In my case, it entirely obliterated it!

Are opportunities more available or is practice more limited because of this new responsibility? And is healthcare to the poor suffering as a result?

The profession finally got out from under the repressive Board of Medicine in the state and allowed regulation to occur from the holistic perspective of the Nursing Board. I can only hope that this will ultimately liberate the role of Nurse Practitioners.

Recent surveys among patients of every demographic show that people value the care given them by Nurse Practitioners over the time constraining limits of doctors, or other specialists. The patients feel that their concerns are being heard, that Practitioners will make the best decisions with the collaboration of all concerned in the healthcare team.

They know that the decisions are based on good medicine, and that all considerations are carefully given the time they deserve.

I used to see between twenty and thirty patients each day. I ordered tests that I used to diligently follow. I kept track of each person, learned about her family members, and kept in mind any trauma she might have been experiencing.

I made sure she was linked to the social service agency who could provide more extensive help

Over half of my patients were children. About every two months, I cared for a child who had been sexually or physically abused.

I remember being called to testify on a child's behalf who lost weight in his mother's care, but thrived with his grandmother. His grandmother was not seeking to take visitation away from his mother and indeed, welcomed the mother's presence in his life.

I could not understand why the case was going to court. The child's mother had never been able to attend to her own needs, got involved with men who beat her, did drugs and always ended up in prison. I felt the court case was a supreme waste of time and money. I broke all the rules of testimony and court etiquette that day and got away with it. Usually, when called to bear witness, one is expected to sit quietly, answer questions only when asked and give objective data that we all hope will be used to save the child from any more distress.

Instead, I stood at the bench, faced the mother and said, "I believe we are wasting everyone's time here, today. It is clear to me that your child should live with his grandmother where he is clothed, fed and given a stable place to live. It is clear that you have had a difficult time providing the same level of protection for this child.

"If you give your grandmother the responsibility to attend to your son, she will want you to help with his care. Your son will best benefit from this arrangement."

I sat down, fully expecting to be reprimanded for this short speech which did not at all follow court protocol.

The lawyers looked relieved, as did everyone else, including the child's mother. That day, the child went home to live with his grandmother.

Not long after, his mother was murdered in her apartment.

The Pediatric Guru brought an enlightened response to the court system regarding child abuse in York, Pennsylvania due to his tireless advocacy of abused children for the last forty years in that town. Police, lawyers and judges no longer turn an eye of denial to these cases.

But recently, a child in my care, five years of age, had been allegedly sexually abused and was the target of a sex ring in another state. The case was held outside of York and was heard in the city where the abuse took place.

The child had been graphic in her descriptions of sexual and physical violence. She told a counselor and a Children and Youth worker about her experiences without any prompting from the adults.

And she ran away from home twice before she was four and one half years of age.

When the case was first heard, the judge was openly agitated by the nature of the case, and was heard to say, "This is no place for a case like this," and the case was subsequently dropped in that town.

The local police never investigated the household where the child had been living.

The child lived in a loving environment with her paternal grandparents, but there was a constant threat that she could go back to live with her mother, who was fighting for custody, and back to the place where she was allegedly forced to wear makeup and dress in stylish clothing and perform oral sex with adults who came as far as New York to sexually abuse her.

The courts handed her back to the perpetrators.

In retrospect, was this a case of Human Trafficking, and we missed it? Had we properly identified the case as Trafficking instead of child sexual abuse, would we have been able to save her from her perpetrators?

We encouraged her to voice her truth, while she was in our care as Health Care Providers, to be the person she is meant to be and to more than survive but to shine in the soul she has been blessed with and is her own to fulfill.

This is not meant in any way to turn away from the brutalities this child has seen and felt. Statistics tell us all about the problems people have who experience sexual and physical violence in early years.

But studies also show that when people are given support, love and an abundance of healing and counseling work, these scars upon the psyche can be channeled towards art and creativity and an appreciation for the great gifts that are available in everyday life.

My work allows me to listen to the stories of many, many people. At the end of any saga, I encourage with a vision to the great potential of the person. My job has given me a sense, a feeling, a knowing of what good a person is capable of achieving.

This, combined with medical knowledge and experience, has created an intuitive approach to people and their problems. I feel in my gut and heart what is needed and what a person could do to be happy. I need to lead them unobtrusively in a direction whereby potential can begin to be realized.

A nurse can go to school for years, master nursing theory, get a PhD, but there is no substitute for working face to face with families, meeting a patient on her own terms and developing relationships that embrace an entire community.

Only the passage of time can teach wisdom borne of experience encompassing trial and error. And even then, there are no guarantees.

I cannot directly teach my students openness towards people, or teach them how to drop all judgement in the face of the seeming mistakes and milestones of our patients, or teach them how to celebrate in the face of it all.

I cannot teach them how to love patients and people other than by example. Even then, they take with them what is needed at the time. Much of what they hear deals with medical protocol but I hope the underlying lessons of humanity become clear, with time.

And in a busy office environment with isolated conversations, ringing phones and lines of people waiting for service, all in a basement without windows that give vision to cloud and sky, it is not surprising that for most of us, the secret meaning of Universal Truth is lost in the 9 to 5 work-a-day world.

Workers do not feel free to discuss what would give them ultimate satisfaction to live out the rest of life with peace of mind. At the end of the work week, nerves are shaken and mundane activities obscure the excitement of the journey as a whole.

We plod along and fail to give our unique gifts to one another. We don't like to acknowledge the constant presence of the unyielding and solemn patriarchy that dominates the medical workplace. This grim wraith that shadows our movements and weighs upon the psyche is tempting to deny and ignore.

This coupled with windowless rooms situated right next to the mortuary causes a morose orientation to life that does not soar with the upward spiral of an eagle in flight. Once we can point to the gestapo that is medicine, that everywhere surrounds us in our career lives and say AHA! I've just named the demon! can we move on to save the world.

Chapter Seven: The Medical Gestapo

As I was growing up, my family doctor was a homeopath who did not believe in childhood immunizations, fluoride in the water or antibiotic therapy. I never took an antibiotic until well after my twentieth birthday. Now my health is robust, surely as a consequence of my childhood homeopathic constitutional remedy.

Homeopathy treats with remedies that stimulate the immune system to work in concert with nature, the tides and the elements to heal the body of illness. Even though I've never really understood one explanation as to how it works; it works from the inside out.

My family doctor was singled out many a time by the Board of Medicine and the American Medical Association for treating people with methods that were not strictly allopathic. He did not recommend chemotherapy or radiation for cancer, or pain killers at the first sign of a headache, unless a person in their belief system wanted these treatments.

But people came to him because they did not want conventional therapies, and felt supported by the doc for their choices. They were searching for a medical approach that sustained and encompassed mind, body and spirit.

My family doctor was continuously harassed by the medical establishment who threatened to take his license because he was not a robot dolling out pills and substances that in truth, do deplete the immune system.

He helped heal cases deemed hopeless by medical science.

My husband, Tom, was so dangerously anemic that the emergency room doctors were arranging for him to have a blood transfusion. This was at a time when the HIV virus was contaminating America's blood supply in the early 1980s.

Tom refused treatment and left the hospital against medical advice.

He paid a visit to the homeopath, a referral made by America's most prolific poet, Ted Enslin. After an hour long history, a history much different than the histories we are taught to do in the traditional medical model, the homeopath gave Tom a remedy that was dispensed under the tongue and dissolved instantly.

In two days, he was able to climb a stairway without collapsing with shortness of breath. Every day, he felt an ever increasing strength he could not deny and his blood iron level was restored in six to eight weeks.

There are many other stubborn people just like Tom who do not want to go to the doctor and be prescribed toxic medicines. They want to be listened to and want a personal experience of true healing when they become ill.

Many people want the opportunity to view their illness as an entry point to spiritual insight, and not have a panicked person treating them who is terrified of death and specifically of their own mortality.

John Robins has perfectly outlined the gestapo of medicine in his articulate book, *Reclaiming Our Health*. I recommend this book to all the free thinkers of the world who are in tune with their bodies and souls and who want some excellent verification for continuing on the pathway called, "Thinking for myself, and glad of it."

Even though complementary practices have nearly reached the medical mainstream–with mind/body centers being sponsored by allopathic institutions, including the hospital where I work-there still is considerable resistance to it, an arrogance on the part of doctors, and many Nurse Practitioners, for that matter.

This arrogance produces a creatively stifling environment.

The pharmaceutical companies have a monopoly on the chemicals that are prescribed and research is only done on the medicines that make the most money for the pharmaceutical cartels.

The Federal Drug Administration, The American Medical Association, The Board of Medicine et al are still hanging on to a rigid scientific, mechanistic view of life that does not support the spirit that moves through all of life- the breathing, constantly renewing out of the ashes mythical perspective that gives meaning to every moment.

I always tell my students, there is another way. People often come to the hospital because of acute conditions that require immediate attention. If all goes well, and being human does not equal making drastic mistakes or oversights, then a person can expect to be helped by allopathic medicine.

Now more than ever, and more so in the future, Registered Nurses and Nurse Practitioners can practice with our hearts and not compromise our values. We'll listen to our patients and make recommendations based on what we know to be true and right.

I'll give alternative treatment advice in regard to Ritalin for ADHD children, to chemotherapy, if a person refuses to have it, to the medicalization of childbirth and menopause, for the people who are open to it.

Woman need to be reminded of their own strength, beauty and resilience and we are in a position to give that to our patients. And not surprisingly, we are given the same empowerment in return.

Yet the gestapo of medicine exists, is all around us and has permeated the collective world view of medicine for over one hundred years. It does no good to deny it. Nurses know better than doctors how to free medicine from the death grip that doctors and their patriarchal organizations have created.

All of us have to see it for what it is and take a stand against the destruction and say we no longer want this in our professional lives which bleeds over into every other aspect of living.

And unbeknownst to doctors at this time, they do not benefit from holding on to organizations that stifle the human spirit. Now it is time to seek another way.

Old ways die hard. Hospitals have become businesses rather than healing centers, becoming victims of corporate takeovers.

The old boy network thrives in this environment, prompting workers in the front lines who deal with the day by day frustrations of failing health in our patients and in the bureaucratic organizations of the workplace-to smell that offending odor of the smoke called Burn Out.

Chapter Eight: Burn Out

I developed a cough in June of 1993 that was persistent and constant. I had a difficult going to work every day, but I did go. I coughed all night long. I no longer could sleep with Tom. I moved a bed to the sun porch with windows over looking a large expanse of sky. I watched the moon move across the heavens from June to early August, all phases of it. Even the conspicuous darkness of the moon, I noticed. I saw the stars shift position throughout the night. I watched the lightening bugs scatter their twinkling light across the pasture and into the leaves of the locust and maple.

One night, I drove myself to the emergency room. The doctor there gave me codeine cough medicine and an antibiotic. I was so sick, I used both medicines. The codeine allowed me to sleep for the first time in weeks.

The Pediatric Guru asked me about the cough, not long after I started the antibiotic. He was sure the cough was Pertussis, or whooping cough. I stood in the clinic hallway, coughing until reaching the end of a breath, then whooped and vomited. He told me, based on the classic presentation of the cough, that there was no doubt about the diagnosis.

Then he and a family practice resident at the time compared information about the patients we recently took care of in the clinic. One was a baby whom I briefly saw and then another resident admitted him into the hospital. He was later diagnosed with Pertussis and died soon after. The child had not received any immunizations.

Adults do not die of whooping cough. The immunizations received in infancy against Pertussis wear off when a person reaches adulthood. I saw in one great moment the wisdom of immunization programs and since that time, have never doubted the services rendered from such public service policies. These policies are a win for allopathic medicine.

The illness wore me down. I did not have the strength to even speak to people without coughing. I recently had been accepted into a program at the hospital called Clinical Pastoral Education. Even though I was not a pastor, I convinced the head of the curriculum that nursing was my ministry.

But the head of the Ob/Gyn department at the time, a man whose solemn face will soon join the unsmiling portraits around the hospital, told me he would not allow me to take the course, since some of the course work cut into my clinical work hours.

The disappointment I felt created an imbalance within my immune system, and a drop in my resistance to disease, allowing the Pertussis to take hold.

I finally took to my bed and lay there for several days, with shallow breath and absolutely no thought to distract me. I saw small colorful dots in my visual field.

Then Tom brought me a piece of mail, inviting me to learn a meditation technique disseminated by Self Realization Fellowship in Los Angeles. I sat up in bed and gazed into the eyes of the picture of Paramahansa Yogananda, the Indian saint who brought this meditation to America.

I found the energy to immediately send for the meditation instruction. Plus, I had some of Yogananda's books, and I put together a meditation to heal my lungs from his writings. I began to do it morning and evening, starting that day.

I was astonished by the results. With in a day, I was out of bed. The cough was subsiding. The eyes of the saint beamed an understanding of love and compassion into my heart I had not previously experienced.

I learned that spiritual practices are the missing link to fathoming how the immune system works. Burn out can be avoided if people consistently turn to the energy of higher understanding in whatever way makes sense to that person.

A general breakdown of mind, body and spirit is inevitable with over work, lack of exercise, consuming bad food, eating a poor diet, smoking cigarettes, doing drugs, drinking alcohol, lack of sleep, acting like a victim and caving in to disappointment.

Love thy neighbor as thyself is a spiritual practice in its simplicity. How can this truth become second nature if loving the self is not openly embraced? Only in healing ourselves can we open to the vital energy of the universe and use that power for all who come to us for help.

Chapter Nine: Time Clock Tyranny

Time clocks are stationed at strategic locations around the hospital for nurses, secretaries, house keeping staff, cafeteria workers and many others. Doctors and Nurse Practitioners do not have to take their mandatory name badges and swipe through upon arrival and departure. But I have watched as workers storm into the hospital at a racing clip, with furrowed brow and eyes that do not express any other desire but to reach that time clock at the specified time.

A nurse told me recently that hospitals are luring new employees to their facilities with money bonuses plus the promise of a house keeper and lawn person to take care of their affairs, presumably as they work even longer hours to make more money.

My response to this was that if the workplace assigned social harmony as its number one priority, whereby workers were encouraged to laugh and have fun, and wanted to arrive to work because of this expansive vibration channeled to unconditional service-- and time clocks were banished for the tyranny that they represent, then that would be enough to lure the people who are looking for an enlightened work environment to come to such a place to work.

The time clock in the basement near the clinic is the size of a small box, with a constant automated reading of the time flashing across the front of it. Around the corner and straight down the hall is the morgue. Everyone in the general vicinity shares the time clock with clinic workers, as well as those who work in physical therapy and occupational medicine, whose offices are down an opposite hallway.

The line up of workers at the time clock when the shift begins show signs of strain after the rush to arrive but also a certain kind of relief borne from the reality of a safe arrival.

At shifts end, the line up is undoubtedly in another kind of hurry, racing ahead to the rest of the day. This mad speed up is an ongoing phenomenon. The time clock encourages a fast-paced, unthinking mind set, whereby to question this barbaric, unhealthy practice of always being on time--whose time? is equal to going up against a fascist dictator. It seems that the worker never dares to question this manner of operation.

If I was required to swipe in at the time clock, I would be the leader of a time clock rebellion. I would organize a time clock hunger strike and workers all through the hospital would do an organized sit-in to protest this obviously unhealthy practice of reporting to a time clock, moments better spent fostering social harmony in the workplace. The time clock box could be transformed to a collection coffer, to feed the hungry in our community.

Only then will the Age of Aquarius officially begin.

PART TWO: Waking Up In the Patriarchal Medical System
Preface

We always dream before we wake up. And even if the dream is unremembered, the dream images inform the way each step is placed in any direction every day of our lives.

One day I awake and remember a dream. All the women who ever occupied the morgue are lined up for miles at the registration window, wrapped as Egyptian mummies, waiting for me to give them an annual pap test and pelvic exam. They are silent. The task before me feels formidable. I know it will take me forever to do all those exams.

I stood in front of the long, endless line and said, "You do not need to have a pap test! You are already dead!"

And they disappeared as tiny flecks of white light, like millions of fairy bells going back to the oceanic flow of eternal life.

Chapter Ten: Mussolinian Leadership

Time clock tyranny generates a leadership style of autocracy, power and control creating an atmosphere of apprehension among the workers. That is what was created in our clinic and until we could propel ourselves out of our denial and name the oppression for what it was. We were lulled into a nightmare of unquestioned acquiesce to an intolerable work environment.

My nurse of eight years recently left our clinic. She felt an invisible hand around her neck squeezing off her will to live. Five other of my close clinic buddies have left for the same reason, before the tightening noose would lock them in a stranglehold.

On her last day of work, my nurse and I went outside for a farewell chat. She told me she felt liberated because she was leaving and no longer had to face our boss who watched every move the staff made. She never gave face-to-face positive feed back as to the great work everyone was doing. The environment was oppressive enough given the windowless ambience and the burning light of fluorescence, never known to cast a clear light of wisdom on the soul of any one person.

Now, it was over, and she was leaving.

She had gotten a job where she was the boss over a small medical staff and could use her natural skills of compassionate leadership to build a medical practice that had been compromised by the oversights of another manager, who was moving on.

And now, the pure oblivion of being without my friends was facing me. I really was going into a dungeon every day, starkly seeing the harshness of illness and emotional imbalance in an unhealing place, without the outlet of a few giggles and knowing glances passed between familiar friends.

Having fun makes a certain kind of boss uncomfortable. If too much genuine laughter is randomly released, she thinks the next step is to push the mouth downward and get back to work. The idea here is that fun and work are mutually exclusive. Fun gets out of hand. Fun leads to the contagion of having more and more fun, making the human being more beautiful to look at.

Women who do not question the patriarchy and believe they must lead without compassion with a stern rule and unsmiling demeanor are sacrificing themselves to the old world paradigms of unyielding rules and regulations. This does not help the institution nor the women who ignore the aspects of themselves that can cry and love and also can be tough, if needed.

Nor does it help the people who punch the time clock nearly everyday of their lives in search of social harmony.

So I have surrounded myself with students. They make me laugh and I can have a free exchange with them about allopathic and complementary medicine, about the dilemma of any one patient and our ability to positively impact their lives. I tell them to arrive to clinical without rushing, and to have fun while they are here.

We discuss Nurse Practitioner politics and the future of medicine in America.

I wish I could have had as much fun in Nurse Practitioner training, but I am making up for it now.

Chapter Eleven: Poverty Medicine

I found a statue of the Sacred Heart in a Roman Catholic cemetery near a local beer micro-brewery, in my hometown.

The statue is the size of a giant and stands looking down at the grave side of a person long at rest. The best way to gaze into the eyes of the compassionate Jesus is to lie on the ground, with another tomb stone as a head rest, and look straight up.

Then and only then do the eyes which have seen all suffering and joy look directly at you, with upraised hands showing the marks of the crucifixion, showering blessings down upon you. The great flame leaping from the heart of the icon gives rise to an other worldly feeling as I lie on the ground, looking up at the healing image that has transformed the world.

I evoked that image and all the other healing images of my life as difficult situations arose in the bowels of the hospital where I used to work, or now, in the Labor and Delivery suite. The time clock audibly ticks away each moment in the bright fluorescence removed from sky and cloud and the song of the bright red cardinal.

And as a Labor and Delivery nurse, the image of Saints, Holy Ones and Angels create a calm within my psyche.

I like to take a cue from those saints who passed before us who took care of the poor, healed the sick, raised the dead. I sometimes imagine our workplaces as a monastary, of sorts, where our mission in life can be carried out. Yet not one of the workers there have taken the vow of charity, poverty or celibacy. Those images of Mother Theresa, Saint Katherine of Drexel, Ghandi, Jesus or the Buddha are unspoken dreams that come to remind us of the nobility of our daily task as we embark on yet another day of poverty medicine.

I want my students to have a sense of purpose, of destiny about their work with patients and their families. This is not an easy concept to discuss or even to instill. It must come from within the person doing the service. Many doctors have written about an initial vision that drove them to pursue medical training. Then at the end of the educational experience the original intent to help and to serve becomes stifled as a coldly mechanized and scientific world view takes its place.

Nurses enter their profession with the same vision of altruistic service. Nursing education is not as long as that of the doctor.

That first intention which was fresh and innocent to begin with can be pieced back together to serve as a map of destiny.

Florence Nightingale is a model for the nursing vision of service and compassionate caring to our patients but so are all the saints who served the poor and healed the sick by the simple power of love. Instead of reading medical journals, I'd like to read aloud to my students the writings of Mother Teresa, the Dalai Lama, of Yogananda or Vivakananda, another great Indian saint. We could pass the book around the circle and take turns reading.

And the grim, unsmiling faces of the patriarchy will fade into the sunrise of a new medical age.

Chapter Twelve: Welfare to Work

The one radical element that has suffered the most in the welfare to work programs all across the nation and can be seen as a casualty-is our children.

The children of the world are everyone's children. The children in my clinic wanted me to see them as my own. I felt a special responsibility towards them. They came to their appointments, mostly smiling and well pleased, sometimes crying in anticipation of the dreaded but necessary immunization. There was a knowing, a freshness and an innocence in their clear eyes that wanted to trust everything about the world and the people in it. But inevitably, this certainty in the goodness of all things does come to an end, with the potential of returning later with spiritual understanding.

I used to like to hold informal surveys among patients who came to me, usually single mothers entering job training programs where wages were low and did not offer health insurance.

They were forced to place their children in day care settings.

When the children got sick and couldn't go to

day care, these mothers needed to stay home, thus threatening their low wage jobs. If family support was nonexistent, these single moms quickly found themselves in a stalemate with their lives. Selling drugs and prostitution must become an all too necessary home-based business.

If the children of the world are not regarded as every mother and father's child, and a separation occurs between an individual and what she is capable of giving to the world, society and to the culture, then a rare opportunity for contribution is gone. The bestowal of every person's gift to the world is a bounty of genius.

I think of the Pediatric Guru and what he would say to this. He, above all else, is a teacher to many. I certainly am one of his more eager students. He would want me to continue to take in more apprentices and would encourage me to show them the importance of their responsibility to the world through their own unique style of patient care. He would want me to appreciate their distinct view of humanity and to encourage discourse on saving the planet for all unborn children.

Recently we sat together at a bar. He sipped a

strong Manhattan with a bright red cherry on top, and I enjoyed my first micro-brewed beer of the week. We spoke of his own life, of his hope to find the love of his life, and of me continuing to work at the clinic after my newly found liberation from the boss, who no longer had any influence over me. We drank to that.

He wanted to know exactly how to tell a person that he wanted to marry them. I told him to get down on his knees so she wouldn't be able to miss the message behind his words. Then we laughed about the possibility of not being to get back up again.

I remember the first day I met the Pediatric Guru. He was interviewing me for the job at the clinic that served the indigent. I had been practicing a breath exercise for weeks before our planned meeting which helps to intensify the energy exchange between people, animals, trees and even rocks. In this instance, the energy flowed between the Guru and me.

It took about five minutes before I felt him relax. I was told that the Guru would be the greatest obstacle to my getting the job. Yet this was no grueling challenge: It was pure fun. When I told him that I'd rather work on an Indian reservation but considered the clinic the second best choice, I knew I had the job by his reaction. He beamed and laughed and ended the interview. He walked me down the stairway and I believed his feet were dancing. I later heard him explain to someone else that I was a person who interviewed well. In reality, we had a heart to heart bond that transcends all explanation.

Hundreds of children have been cared for by P. Guru over the years. His children patients, now grown, look back at the encouragement they received from him and know his influence made them who they are in this moment, often in the face of broken and violent homes, alcoholism and drug addiction. He never turned anyone away for care. He saw them all as his family. That is the legacy he has given to all of us who know him now or have ever known him.

Chapter Thirteen: Inspired Living versus Loss of Vision

When my aunt turned ninety, I asked her to explain what she attributed to her longevity and lucidity of thought. She said simply, "...to my ability to rest when I am tired. I've done that every day of my life."

She recently passed on at 102.

Aha! I thought, knowing when to stop, and to resume again when feeling fresh and enthusiastic, and not imposing my rhythms on anyone else, or thinking someone else's cycle must be my own. Viewing each day as an art form that constantly evolves and changes, and when nearing the end of life, knowing when the creation of my life has reached a dimension where someone else can pick it up and integrate what I've learned into her unfolding creative life.

I made an expressive statement to a group of women with whom I work, all in their fifties, as we were drawing up shots to give to unsuspecting children. I said that soon I was going to turn fifty and I was excited because, the way I saw it, our mid-life years are an opportunity for growth and expansion.

I was nearly booed out of the room.

I said, "I've never felt better in my life." The women grumbled and left the room with shots in hand.

I was amazed. How can anyone possibly think that fifty is old, or any other age, really, if we actively pursue the energy of each day and use it, mold it and rest with it as we feel the ebb and flow from within our souls reflect that which outwardly manifests experience?

I now have a student who will be with me for the next twelve months. Her name is Martha. She will turn sixty as our time together draws to a close. She has been a labor and delivery nurse for over twenty years in inner city Baltimore. Her courage in returning to school at what the world considers to be an advanced age, at retirement, is a testament to thinking big and obliterating ageist philosophies. And she is having a great time doing it.

Martha said to me the other day, "I constantly ask myself why I am doing this, Kate."

And I asked, "Why are you doing it?"

"Because I want to," and that is enough for all of us and for the world she will someday continue making contributions to.

People like Martha are living examples of vitality for women who think they have one foot in the grave at age sixty. She did demonstrate pelvic tilt to a twenty year old pregnant woman one day and developed sciatica over the next weekend. She showed up to clinical the next following week, laughing about the malady.

I decided I would have Martha and a student named Sandy, another Practitioner with great potential and courage, accompany me into the exam room of a fourteen year old boy whose school nurse had diagnosed head lice earlier that day. She sent him to us for the standard treatment.

I said, "What brings you here today, George?" He mumbled something incomprehensible.

Sandy said, with gravity, "Cancer?" because that is what she thought he said.

I said, "Head lice?"

And Martha said, not missing a beat, "I'd rather have head lice any day than cancer."

I know George was not finding any of this to be funny, but we finally broke him down–at least, for a smile.

Chapter Fourteen: Daily Work as Meditation

Simple, repetitive tasks done hundreds of times in the course of a single week give rise to a flow, a taking off with breath and steps into what can be best described as the foundation for spiritual practice. Walking a hall's length, washing hands, drawing up shots, doing physical exams: the more these tasks are repeated, the greater the opportunity to slip into a revelry associated with rhythm, comradery and contact with people.

Staying fully engaged in the moment with a concentration on breathing in and breathing out cuts out mind wandering, distractions and anxiety. Shallow breathing shoots the mind directly into an anxious state.

This does not mean that suddenly all will be well as soon as a meditation practice is taken up, and obstacles will instantly be taken from our path. I recently read a quote by a Tibetan lama, Chogyam Trunga Rinpoche: "Hold the sadness and the pain of samsara in your heart and at the same time the power and vision of the Great Eastern Sun. Then the warrior can make a proper cup of tea."

It seems we think that by concentrating on the power and vision of the Great Eastern Sun, all pain will disappear. But both the sadness that accompanies compassion and the vision of spiritual oneness with all beings everywhere must be held simultaneously in each moment. Then and only then will the task at hand be truly an art form, an authentic expression of who we are in this life time.

To fully engage in each moment, the task at hand becomes a ceremony, an offering that goes straight to the heart of heaven, to all that we envision as right and good. Each simple step, breath and activity becomes an expression of our appreciation for all of life. I watch my dog, Mukunda, as he lives out his day. He bounds forth with a laugh and a growl, always seeing the potential for play in each moment. In this way, he takes his ball where ever he goes, into nursing homes, to picnics, into crowds of children swinging high, and rolls the ball forward to any one as his gift. He sees this as his job in life. He takes his play seriously, and play and work become one.

The reality must be faced: even if I could take Mukunda down into the enclosed space of fluorescence without one glimmer of natural light, how long would he thrive in that environment? The enclosure of walls and floors made entirely of cement has removed any sense of sharing the day full of rhythm marked by the sun's passage, by birdsong and the cawing of the crow.

Mukunda would tell me not to endure this way of life-boxed and confined with artificial barriers. He would tell me that many creatures, when captured and put in zoos, will first die in the face of such confinement.

But here we are anyway-doing time, going into workplaces that separate us from the planetary dance. When the prisoners come to us for care, I realize I am not so far from where they involuntarily spend each day. But I've chosen my place in the world.

I do feel the flow of each step, each breath and the pain inherently connected with doing work in an imperfect world.

Chapter Fifteen: Transforming the Battleground

It is official! Our clinic is moving to a newly built health care facility, six blocks further into the city where most of our patients live. There are windows that span all the way around the building! I refuse to suppress the joy I will feel as a sunray filters through the window, or a flock of geese chances over the building, or a lone pigeon rests upon a window ledge-hopefully the very window where I write on a patient's chart, or in a notebook with a blank white page.

Heaven and hell are in the mind. We take ourselves from the basement bowels to a light filled health care facility. Who is to say that the selves we take with us will be transformed and enlivened by the new space, by the natural light, by the bright fresh colors on the newly built walls? How long will it take before we fall back asleep, stop noticing our surroundings? How can we stay awake?

The trick is to drop the mask and become our true selves, striving to express the joy and sorrows we feel, not what we think others want us to feel. The trick is to move away from the limitations of experience and beliefs that put us in a prison box. The move to our new community health care center is an opportunity to shed the old skin of unauthentic living and move forward with an open and fun filled spirit.

Yesterday, I was told the move has been postponed. I felt like a prisoner who had been told my court hearing for release had been canceled. The ax fell on the vision of freedom that in my mind, fantasized coming out of a dark dungeon into the beautiful sun and cloudless blue sky, feeling natural warmth and coolness on my face with soft breezes lifting my steps to the tree tops.

But the future move-is in the future. I tell myself that no matter what happens, the present moment is the only time there is. Patience can only be learned by slowing down, accepting limitations on time, and allowing the full spectrum of experience to wash through the soul-not next week, but now.

The battleground, the resistance to life, is in the mind. The first response is to resist, the ego's response, then when guidance is sought in silence, whole worlds of wisdom arise to dispel the myth of duality, the great illusion that separates me from everyone and everything else in the universe.

So the resistance must be acknowledged, moved through, and in a quiet state, transformed to that of peace.

Today, I go back to the clinic basement. I will do there today what I've done every day for the past ten years which is to first of all show up, feel good and attend to the myriad tasks at hand. I will speak to one hundred people during the course of the day, and put all of my natural enthusiasm into the tone of my voice. I will smile at people. I will gaze at the picture of my dog on the way to the fax machine.

And all will be right with the world.

Chapter Sixteen: Merging Allopathic and Complementary Medicine

It is 1995 and Tom's mentor and teacher, Leonard Laskow, is coming to town. He is author of *Healing With Love* and Tom is completing the certification program in Holoenergetic Healing, the healing model outlined in the book.

I boldly tell Dr. Laskow that I will arrange for him to talk to the residents one morning and then to open the auditorium at the hospital to the community that same evening in 10/95. I figure that since he is an Ob/Gyn physician that I may be able to follow through with my promise.

The biggest hurdle is to get clearance from the then head of the Ob/Gyn department, Dr. Lamone, who is the most scientific, allopathic person I have ever known. I first secure Dr. Laskow's visit with the Behavioral Health and Oncology Departments, whom agree to jointly sponsor this event.

When I finally ask Dr. Lamone for his support for the program, he put me off a few days, then hesitantly acquiesces. He realizes that the event has already gained momentum and he would look like a smuck if he tried to block it now.

So it is a Go! But a rocky go with Dr. Lamone, who I believe in the back of his mind realizes that patients want information on Complementary Medicine and, indeed, at that time in 1995, over one third of all consumers in America had tried at least one complementary therapy. He knows that the physician community must acknowledge and respect people's choices–or else they will lose all of their patients!

But my enthusiasm for what was rapidly becoming a happening and a party was getting on Dr. Lamone's nerves. I advertised the event in the hospital's weekly newspaper and the local newspaper and I used the employee wide computer communication system to tell people to come to the event. I sent out a mass mailing. I raised several thousand dollars from different pharmaceutical companies and the hospital also gave one thousand dollars to sponsor the good doctor.

Finally a few days before the affair, Dr. Lamone came to my office and shut the door. He had a copy of *Healing With Love* in his hand and he hurled it across the room. I backed up and it narrowly missed my head!

I said, "Are we having a bad day today, Sir!" trying to sound like a military officer. I laughed then, thinking that using the book as a weapon was the last application Dr. Laskow had in mind for his book.

He made a few threats about my boldness but quickly gave up because I was having such a good time.

=--=-=-=-=-=-=-

Sam was dying of colon cancer. He saw the small ad in the York paper for the Laskow occasion and a small but persistent voice from within his psyche told him to look a second time-and come to the community gathering at the hospital.

I saw Sam come to the auditorium on the arm of his wife. He was short of breath and had a greyness to his skin and face. Tom and I immediately welcomed and sat with them during Dr. Laskow's talk and presentation. Sam told us his story. He said his doctors did not give him long to live. I asked him if he would like a personal healing session scheduled with the doctor. He indicated without hesitation that he would.

We kept in touch with Sam after our first meeting and for the two years until his death. After the Holoenergetic work he did with Laskow, work that stimulates the body's own immune system to repair itself, Sam's energy returned, the serum levels that signify an acute condition gradually decreased and he was able to complete the unfinished business he felt he needed to settle with his family. Soon before he died, he told us he was ready to die.

It is the year 2000. We now have what is called the Mind/Body Center affiliated with the hospital just a five minute walk down the street. The Center offers a wide range of complementary therapies. Tom has completed his training as a Holoenergetic Practitioner, and will start work at the Mind/Body Center as an independent contractor in 2001. This would not have been possible ten or even five years ago.

Dr. Lamone has retired and a woman physician has taken his place. I wonder if her portrait at retirement time will be the first female picture to brighten the grim suit and tie line up throughout the hospital hallways? I wonder if the institution as we know it will even exist in fifty years as all people and creatures will be equal under the sun, standing on firm ground and green grass with the consciousness that anything is possible?

Chapter Seventeen: Pathological Optimism

I was preparing a talk for a recent staff meeting entitled: "Learned Optimism," based on the work of Martin Seligman, famous for his work on happiness, optimism, pessimism and learned helplessness. The whole point of the talk was that optimism is a better lens through which to view the world. It stimulates the immune system and makes for a more congenial approach to life.

I was going to give the staff a quiz to determine if the people there had a natural leaning towards an optimistic or pessimistic explanatory style. Then I was going to give insights as to how each person could change her world view if she tended to be more pessimistic. I would explain how an optimist sees unfortunate life events as temporary and surmountable: as challenges to be overcome.

The pessimist sees set backs that happen to them as permanent and insurmountable. They blame themselves for all personal unfortunate life circumstances. This way of viewing the world leads to feeling helpless, with depression often an inevitable result.

I believed this made perfect sense. But

suddenly I was gripped with a hesitancy about giving the staff this kind of material when they have to punch a time clock twice a day with fluorescent glare burning the eyes. They have to bear a boss who is rarely forthcoming in her appreciation of what the staff contributes on a daily basis. I felt the talk was furthering a message already well positioned in the patriarchal organization of not saying how you feel, of smiling when sad, of forcing a phony veil over reality.

I thought about positive thinking in the workplace. The boss opens every meeting by going around the room and asking everyone to say a good word about what happened to them that month as a result of another staff member. People's voices sound a note or two above their normal tone as goody two shoes takes over their persona, giving an example of a good deed done by a fellow co-worker. No one wants to go to these meetings, but they must because they are mandatory.

I had heard about a memo every secretary received who worked in the emergency room. It warned against the expression of any negativity. If anything of a negative nature was reported to or heard by an administrative power, then the person responsible for these words was in jeopardy of losing her job. Furthermore, every secretary of that department was required to wear a hospital polo shirt, tucked in to mandatory white nurses pants. No discussions about individual preferences were allowed.

Positive thinking seen in this light is only for upholding the status quo at the expense of an individual who may have feelings of unrest and dissatisfaction, yet is not permitted to express them or anything else in this climate where enforced happiness is the rule.

If a poll was conducted, asking how many people take an antidepressant just to be able to tolerate the dysfunctional climate of enforced happiness, where no one is permitted to say how they feel, or to cry, I would hazard a guess that almost every worker takes it, or wishes they were taking it, or will be taking it soon. If these same people were involved in a pursuit that stimulated passion and inspiration every day, where some financial success was realized in a flexible daily schedule, then antidepressants would no longer be necessary.

I abandoned the talk on "learned optimism" and no longer go to staff meetings. I have a few extra hours to write these words in my kitchen with a sturdy slate grey ceramic tile floor under my feet that Tom and I laid down last summer. Mukunda lies to my left. It is all Saints Day and the sky is a deep blue in the dawning of another day. The pasture is still green. The river that runs past our house has leaves scattered across her surface. I hear a bird giving an introductory greeting to this stunning crisp autumn gift of a day: Another moment free of fluorescence and stale office air.

Chapter Eighteen: Advocacy

The crowded office I share with four other women has become loud with ringing phones, two or three at once. Secretaries walk in and out at regular intervals, asking questions about patients who have called or shown up feeling ill and asking to be seen immediately.

The business day takes off and suddenly we realize that we did not drink a drop of water all day, or take a lunch, or go outside and walk in the natural light. We did not go to our car parked next to a tree to relax or meditate in the noon day sun. In short, we have failed to advocate for ourselves. Too many more days like this and we won't be able to advocate for anyone else, either.

We walk into the bowels of the hospital basement in the dark of early morning hours of winter and do not leave until long after the sun has gone down. We are dehydrated and hungry from eating on the run if eating has taken place at all, nerves drained from too many conversations with too many people.

I long ago abandoned nursing co-dependency and decided without doubt that if I don't take care of myself, no one else will do it for me. I take for myself stolen moments from each day to do sitting meditation in my car parked next to a tall and hearty oak or maple tree. I drink plenty of water, minimize talking or go to another part of the hospital and talk to other employees whom I have never met before.

I also see all of my patients, plus a few others, besides. Each day has its own rhythm as do our bodies and spirits. We must listen to our feelings, to our cells and always ask, periodically, "Do I need to slow down, to go inwardly to the God within for the rest needed to enjoy a peaceful moment?"

We cannot be true advocates for our patients until we love ourselves, first. I remember when I was in nursing school, for the first round, getting an Associates degree in nursing in Corvallis, Oregon. I remember one of our preceptors of whom all the student nurses spoke reverentially. She was, they said, a patient advocate.

What did that mean, exactly? It meant different things, depending on whom I'd ask.

One person cited her diligence in taking care of patients. She took time to be with them, thus staying late to complete her charting.

Another person was focused on this woman's outspoken qualities, in that she formed patient advocacy committees, and was on the forefront of keeping costs down. She encouraged patient feedback so that what was suggested was implemented.

In my current Labor and Delivery nursing position, patients are ecstatic about the care they receive. If I see a woman with a newborn in public, I'll ask the new mom where she had the baby.

She invariably says "The Women and Babies Hospital," because no one wants to deliver anywhere else.

And when I say I work there, the woman becomes enraptured and lovingly describes her care she received from everyone she contacted, the nursing staff in particular.

At the heart of this is a dedication to patient care and a loyalty to our patients. When the nurses have a few moments, we sit and talk about our patients. We describe her labor progress and if the doctor or mid-wife is off or on in the care they are giving, we discuss that with each other, too.

The nurses are a cohesive group. We have a

bond that can be described as a sister-hood. We have to be close, I've found, because the doctors and midwives, in most cases, do not support us as equals. They speak to us as if we were servants.

This doesn't fly with women who expect to be treated as equal partners with respect-as we all need to be treated-but often realize, sadly, that we will not be.

Unless there is a massive consciousness raising.

Nurses and Nurse Practitioners must advocate for our patients. We pray: anyone who comes before us today seeking help will find it by our diligence in breaking through the barriers that obstruct the process, at this time. We hope to listen without judgement, with a calmness that springs from our ability to love ourselves as much as the person standing before us, now. We do this in the spirit of all who have been our teachers and our loving ability to be teachers to those who still want to be Nurses. We do this in the faith that all will flow in the current of connection with those who come to us today and everyday, that they find the help they are looking for.

Om Peace Amen.

Chapter Nineteen: Work Place Diversity

Nurses are mostly white and mostly women. Nursing is about to become obsolete as a profession.

The nursing shortage may not remedy itself this time as it has in the past. Women have greater career options available to them now and can choose to enter any field, get better salaries, not work mandatory overtime as so many nurses do today. It is not appealing to the woman of today to answer to the predominately white male profession of physicians who have some serious soul searching to do regarding their attitudes towards women and nurses in particular.

The mean age of the average nurse today is forty-five. After retirement age in another twenty years, the elderly people in this country will be facing a depletion of skilled health care and at the same time the aging baby boomers as a population will outnumber the younger generations. We must remedy this problem now or we will face a serious health care crisis in the next twenty years.

The nursing profession must undergo a massive consciousness raising if it hopes to survive the twenty-first century.

Who are we, as the white women who dominate the nursing profession? Who do we want to become? Why doesn't our profession appeal to a wider diversity of multi cultural people, both men and women?

The answer lies in exploring institutional racism as it applies to healthcare in our country today. Do we believe in the myth that America is a white nation that is becoming more diverse and that our goal in healthcare is to help these diverse others be like us?

Do we want our nurses and doctors to strictly adapt the protocols of the AMA, the American Cancer Society and the Board of Medicine, all run on the white paradigm of the status quo and the white male patriarchy?

The allopathic medical model has only recently opened itself to holistic and folk medicine practices, allowing these ideas to be integrated into health care strategies. But chemotherapy, surgery, radiation and antibiotics take priority whenever serious health problems arise. Some people do not want these interventions.

If our patients come to us and want another viewpoint and our support as they explore other options, and all we give them is statistical proof that their choice may lead to an early death without compassion or warmth, then it is obvious that our professions will remain white and our patients will decide never to visit a doctor, nurse practitioner, nurse midwife or physician's assistant again.

We must also explore the white privilege afforded us by our mostly white professions and by the society and culture established after white European immigrants systematically killed the Native American peoples. This is not an exercise for feeling shame for being white. Rather, if the status quo is never questioned and we continue to mindlessly conform to the rules and regulations that are culturally based on white domination, supremacy and racism, then the nursing profession will never survive. In fact, how can any profession survive if people do not move beyond the cultural assumptions that form the foundation of white privilege in America?

Our clinic has moved to a gorgeous new medical arts building in the neighborhood where our patients live. The whole second floor is ours and is comprised of one large expansive window. I fondly called our old digs "the third world clinic." But now, we make up the largest medical group not only of the hospital but of the state serving the most patients, comprised of people on welfare or coming off welfare or who do not have medical insurance. Many patients prefer our care to other doctor's offices, coming to us out of choice with medical insurance that could be taken by any other physician.

The move was not an easy one, especially for the white staff. Fear of being killed in the parking lot after dark by roving black or Hispanic gangs was heard in whispers in the first days of operation. Yet our parking lot became a playground for neighborhood kids after dark. They rode scooters and bicycles, did wheelies with exact precision, especially for the benefit of the persons exiting the building at night. I marveled at their dexterity and ability to entertain.

These children were my patients. They wanted to show all of us the free and boundless spirit we needed to harmonize with in order to provide the best care for them when they graced the exam room for medical care.

We made our move precisely at the time that a local grand jury was wrapping up its investigation into the unsolved murders of an

African American woman and a white police officer during a race riot in the city over thirty years ago. The then mayor of the town was implicated in the murder of Lilly Bell Allen, the young woman who was killed by members of two roving white gangs whose expressed purpose was to kill a person of color during the riot.

The mayor, a police officer at the time, stood up at a rally of all white people, one day before Allen's murder, and shouted "white power," by his own admission. He is being accused of, but denies being the person, who supplied the ammunition that killed the young woman.

Meanwhile, a white police officer lay in a coma at our hospital after being shot driving in the back seat of a tank, proceeding to the scene of another shooting of a white man blasted off his motorcycle by a group of African American men, according to the cyclist. The motorcyclist survived and recently gave his story to the newspaper after many years of pained silence.

In fact, numerous recent newspaper stories chronicle people's memories of the town and their experiences during that riot week. People tell of the town before the riot when black neighborhoods were held hostage by white police officers roving the streets with German Shepard dogs. They attacked man, woman and child at the order of the man in uniform. One of the African American men recently interviewed by the local newspaper rolled up his shirt sleeve and showed the reporter the scars of such an attack.

Everyone agrees that York, PA is not the same town now as it was back then. The grand jury indicted the mayor for the murder of Lilly Belle Allen after he won the local Democratic party run-off election, just days after his victory. But the traumatic memories have resurfaced, and need to be transformed.

The national press has been captured by this story and came to town to do a segment for a nationally televised show. At the same time in the world news was the trial and conviction of a white man found guilty in the 1963 bombing of the Sixteenth Street Baptist Church that killed four African American children in Birmingham, Alabama some thirty-eight years ago.

Our basement clinic now is serving patients in the middle of this controversy, no longer operating in the hospital bowels next to hissing steam pipes, no longer surrounded by the unsmiling portraits of white male doctors lining every entrance way and hallway throughout the institution. The paintings that now adorn our walls are of African American and Hispanic women and their children or of water landscapes situated somewhere in Mexico, Africa or South America.

Some of the children in the parking lot are scratching employee cars and releasing air out of employee tires. So Mukunda the dog and I played Air Bud with the children of the parking lot. We kicked the ball straight into the air and Mukunda leaped to meet it, bouncing the ball off his needle nose. As we played and the children stopped to hug and bring him water, I looked up at the Medical Arts building. It is a beautiful structure, as compared to the falling down homes behind a newly constructed wooden fence, where the children went to fetch a bucket of water to cool off the dog.

And our goal is to deliver the best Allopathic medical care in America. But I realized that the mostly white staff is not seen much out on the street except to walk briskly from their car to the facility. I felt a chill as I realized that we exist in an Ivory Tower. The children and the neighbors think that is also where we exist.

Mukunda and I may have changed that

perception just one small millimeter in the direction of an open embrace of all children everywhere. And Mukunda is not a Pit Bull. His Golden Retriever mixture has given him a loving acceptance of the human condition.

The following week, we pick up Mukunda's companion, Ulysses, a vibrant Golden Retriever puppy. The three of us practiced Play and Peace with the children in our new neighborhood, long after the last clinic session of the day.

Chapter Twenty: National Health Insurance in America

President Clinton and President Bush did not and now President Obama will not address health care reform in a way that deviates even slightly from the HMO, Managed Care and Health Insurance Industries that have given large sums of money to every campaign to keep them quiet. Thus these special interests maintain the status quo of the for profit health insurance corporations that have taken over the health care system in America.

Every day, approximately 100,000 people lose health insurance coverage in the United States. Almost 50 million Americans do not have health insurance at all. The people who have HMO's as their only choice of insurance routinely face rejection of payment when serious health problems arise. The doctors employed by HMO's make decisions about a person's health without laying hands on the patient. They do not examine, listen to or have any contact with the patient about whom life and death decisions are made regarding their health.

This is a human rights abuse in a civil society such as ours, or any other society, for that matter.

There are over 1500 insurance companies in America with different rules of what services will or will not be funded. Our facility has hired two people just to handle the health insurance questions that arise every day. They often have a frustrated and perplexed look in their eyes as they undertake to find solutions to problems, and then have to contact a faceless bureaucratic entity about whether or not a service will be paid for.

Health care providers must also take the time to speak to these people, to convince them to pay for proposed services. Letters must be written to convince the HMO/Managed Care bureaucrats to take a second look at what needs to be done for patients, to ensure good quality medical care.

Health care workers have accepted the unacceptable and do not seem to know the way out of the quagmire.

I recently helped to raise $3,000.00 for a seven year old patient who was in an automobile accident, and suffered a lower spinal cord injury. He is paralyzed from the waist down. The proposed goal for the fund raiser was to buy a handicapped accessible van. Since these vans cost anywhere from $15-30,000.00 dollars, the family bought a computer, instead, enrolled the boy in a study offered online by the Shriner's Hospital in Philadelphia for spinal cord injured patients.

At the fund raising dinner, I sat with the patient's grandmother. She told me she wanted the money to be put in a trust fund to pay for the child's catheter supplies, diapers and medicine that the Managed Care Insurance company would not pay for.

"Wait a minute," I said. "You mean you are paying for all of the supplies out of pocket without insurance reimbursement?"

"Yes," she said.

Back in the office the following week, one of the women whose job it is to deal with insurance questions solved the dilemma and the supplies are now paid for. The child's mother had receipts, and the HMO reimbursed her from the time of the car accident.

I wondered why the insurance company did not automatically pay for these services ? If I had not helped stage an elaborate fund raising event and had dinner with the boy's grandmother, this revelation may not have surfaced. A Universal Single Payer health care plan would make it possible for all people to get the services they need and free up doctors and nurses to give the care that people deserve, plus fulfill all of the reasons doctors and nurses entered their respective professions to begin with: to be of service, to help other people and to bring healing to patients and their families.

National Health Insurance, if implemented, would minimize any disruption to the current health system because health care delivery mechanisms would remain in place while only the financing mechanism changed. Single Payer National Health Insurance would resolve virtually all of the major problems facing America's health care system, today.

Single Payer Insurance is defined as a single government fund with each state paying hospitals, physicians and other health care providers, thus replacing the current multi-payer system of private insurance companies and other plans.

It would provide coverage for the fifty million people who are uninsured.

It would eliminate the financial threat and impaired access to care for tens of millions who do not have coverage and are unable to afford the out-of-pocket expenses because of deficiencies in their insurance plans.

It would return to the patient free choice of health care provider and hospitals, not the choice that only the restrictive health plans allow.

It would relieve businesses of the administrative hassle and expense of maintaining a health benefits program.

It would remove from the health care equation the middleman—the managed care industry—that has broken the traditional doctor-patient relationship, while diverting outrageous amounts of patient care dollars to their own coffers.

It would control health care inflation through constructive mechanisms of cost containment that improve allocation of our health care resources, rather than controlling costs through an impersonal business ethic that robs patients of care so as to increase profits for the privileged few. Single Payer Universal Health Care would provide access to high quality care for everyone at affordable prices. This would be beneficial for individual business as well as the government. So why don't we have a

National Single Payer Plan?

The political will has not gained momentum on this issue due to AMA propaganda that continues to cast doubt in the public mind concerning the success of such a plan. The first misgiving usually offered is that our country cannot afford to pay for comprehensive care for everyone.

Every other industrialized nation provides comprehensive care to all at a much lower cost than our system which leaves so many people out. Other nations spend 6-10 percent of their Gross Domestic Product, or GDP, whereas we, the wealthiest nation on earth, spend 17.9 % of our GDP, in 2011.

Our country already has enough funds dedicated to health care to provide the highest quality of care for everyone. Studies conducted by the Congressional Budget Office, the General Accounting Office, the Lewin Group and Boston University School of Public Health have shown that under a single payer system, comprehensive care can be provided for everyone without spending any more funds than are now being spent. There has been considerable publicity about the delays in receiving elective services that are characteristic of other nations, especially the United Kingdom and Canada. At 6% and 9% of their GDP, respectively, they are spending much less than we are as a nation.

Not only do we have more than sufficient funds, we are also a nation that is infamous for our excess health care capacity. Typical of these excesses is the fact that there are more MRI scanners in Orange County, CA than in all of Canada.

With our generous funding and the tremendous capacity of our health care delivery system, the delays would not be a significant limiting factor in the U. S. "Americans do not want socialized medicine," is a phrase that is frequently used glibly to dismiss the single payer concept. Socialized medicine is a system in which the government owns the facilities, and the providers of care are government employees.

In sharp contrast, a single payer system uses the existing private and public sector health care delivery systems, preserving private ownership and employment. The unique feature of a single payer system is that all health care risks are placed in a universal risk pool, covering everyone. The pool is funded in a fair and equitable manner so that everyone pays their fair share in taxes, unlike our current defective system in which some pay far too much while others are not paying their share. The funds are allocated through a publically administered program resulting in optimum use of our health care dollars.

A single payer system has no more in common with socialized medicine than our current Medicare program.

Many contend that government bureaucracies are very wasteful compared with the efficiencies of the private market place. In the health care arena, this has not been true. Our Medicare program, a publicly administered program, operates on an administrative cost of less than 2%. The managed care intermediaries consume 9 to 30% of the health care dollar.

This difference is due to large corporate administrations, costs involved with competition between companies and marketing expenses that would be nonexistent in a public program. A single payer system has as its mission the optimization of resources for better patient care. Funds are not wasted on corporate administrative excesses.

Another argument is that a single payer system, by being universal, would lower the standard of care to a level of mediocrity for everyone, preventing the affluent from exercising her/his option to obtain the highest level of care.

However, our current system is characterized by essentially two alternatives: either no insurance with severely impaired access to even a mediocre level of care, or being insured by a managed care industry that has whittled down what is available until mediocrity has become the standard of care. Only the relatively affluent have access to unlimited care.

The generous level of funds that we have already dedicated to health care, adding to this a more efficient administration with an exclusive mission of optimum patient care well above the mediocrity that we now have, lays the foundation for a universal health care system in America.

A single payer system does not preclude the affluent from paying, outside the system, for a penthouse suite in the hospital, or for cosmetic surgery or for any other service that should not be part of a publicly funded program.

Other than the assurance that everyone would have coverage for health, there is even a greater good that a single payer system would bring to our nation: Making preventative and public health services available to everyone would improve the level of health of this country. Reduction of communicable diseases and reducing the higher costs of untreated chronic diseases helps us all.

Healthy people, for instance, make for a healthier work force with less lost work time, greater productivity and a more positive healthy environment.

Socialism is a dirty word in this country. Universal health care for all has been equated with socialism, and much propaganda has been communicated by the press, by right wing politicians, by medical groups such as the AMA or anyone else who has an agenda to keep the 1500 plus health insurance companies a thriving market with profits that undoubtedly help to pay for their agendas.

But if Americans knew the truth, and would turn off their TVs and use that time instead to change this country, using the power of grassroots politics, to make a single payer universal system a reality for all, then we would finally have the best health care system in the world. The Green Party in this country has as one of its missions to bring a universal system of health care to all Americans. Any group with the passion to change the world, one issue at a time, with a loving intent, can do it.

I am sure it is only a matter of time.

Chapter Twenty-One: Flow and Resilience and Ecstatic States of Mind

The move from the hospital basement to the corner of South George and Boundary Avenue took many years of planning before the building was raised and finished, and operations began anew. The new medical director was a man with an uncompromising vision of integrity, whose standards of good medical care are unequaled and who probably was a religious saint in a former life. His name here is Dr. Z.

So to think we would just be moving all of the old baggage including our old unchanged selves, and start seeing patients like we always did before, was simply not Dr. Z's plan for us as we began work in the new center.

The first few weeks of the enterprise, to bring better medical access to the indigent of York, Pennsylvania, did not go well. We had no time to unpack before the start of the next scheduled clinic at 8 a.m. Monday morning after a move that took the entire previous weekend. We could not find anything. People who were normally serene with an even temperament began to snap angrily and make demands.

The electrical system failed in the middle of an evening clinic, and the fire alarms went off three times that first week of operation, bringing total building evacuation each time. Rocket Red fire engines appeared but the only fire was in each one of us, unexpressed inner tumult at so much sudden change. But after I took a planned vacation and came back, a reordering of the vibrational fields had taken place and the staff and patient visits were moving along with more courtesy and grace.

Dr. Z. held a space for nourishment of the genius of his staff. In his presence, we felt that he believed in us and we moved more quickly into the manifestation of ever greater potential. This is why he is a great leader. But, the old ways and systems must be redefined. Old leadership styles have outlived their usefulness yet still are used as models. This undermines the organization's ability to be a prototype of excellence for the state of Pennsylvania and the nation.

The Ob/Gyn resident staff continued to conduct a reign of terror on nurses, Nurse Practitioners, secretaries and medical record staff, treating us like a subhuman species with brains the size of a pebble.

The nursing shortage has become a national emergency. If we lose all the nurses, the bedrock foundation of the entire health care delivery system will collapse. The doctor/nurse relationship has long been characterized by condescending attitudes on the part of doctors towards nurses with nurses then repressing feelings of powerlessness. The new breed of nurse is not in the mood to be spoken to or treated in any way other than with respect and civility.

The new breed of doctor, like Dr. Z., would never think of treating anyone unkindly.

But will there be a new breed of nurse? The possibility is significant that no one will replace our current population of retiring nurses. Some young women of today may choose nursing as a career, only to leave it when they see the outdated ways in which women are still expected to perform: groveling before male and female doctors, and tolerating sexual harassment in the process.

Unless we refuse to put up with the put downs, and refuse to tolerate behavior that in the end stifles creativity, making teamwork and flow that can only materialize in harmony impossible, then we will lose our nurses.

According to Mihaly Csikszentmihalyi, flow is the enjoyment of an activity for its own sake. What most matters is not the result of an activity, but the level of control one has acquired over one's attention. When heart, will and mind are synchronized, flow results. Full immersion in an activity is what is required in order for flow to take over. Flow tends to occur when a person faces a clear set of goals that require appropriate responses in order to get a task done. One can consciously create flow experiences by channeling daily activities that produce flow and decrease those that don't.

The work environment is where the majority of flow experiences occur. Incidences of flow can be increased if everyone feels valued and communication between coworkers and their superiors and subordinates are encouraged. The more that teamwork if fostered, where everyone is investing psychic energy into a joint goal, the better will be the environment for flow to occur where greater amounts of creativity are used, and greater degrees of harmony are experienced in the workplace.

Climbing mountains, meditating for three days and joining in sports activities not only open the potential for flow, but also for higher ecstatic states of consciousness.

As a labor and delivery nurse, I have experienced ecstatic states of mind when a baby enters this realm of existence. I can sense the angels, higher guides and the entire ancestral realm as the ultimate support system of the Universe.

Or when my mother died and several of us mid-wived her into the next realm of consciousness-I felt nothing but Love for everything and everyone for many days. This state of mind I am learning to draw on, by the use of imagination and will.

"The important thing is not to think much but to love much; and so do that which best stirs you to love." Saint Teresa of Avila Interior Castle

Love is the ultimate ecstatic state-also joy, the experience of peace and transcendent periods of silence and no thought. Yes we return to ordinary realms of mind, where competition and resentments dominate people's thought forms. Yet once the ecstatic state is achieved-just once-we are never the same again.

We are in the world, not of the world.

Chapter Twenty-Two: The Art and Science and Medicine

Twenty-eight years ago, as I was preparing for my nursing career, I wrote about what I wanted to do and be in order to become the health care provider of my highest ideal. And reading it now, I agree that my ideals in that regard have not changed at all.

First of all, I knew I had to be true to myself in my work as well as all areas of my life. I carefully thought about the science of medicine which fell into the category of rational thinking, ideas proven with good research, as well as the things that are experienced with all five senses. The science of medicine deals with proven facts and dislikes surprises.

The art of medicine falls into the creative medium through which all things are possible, in this existence and beyond. But first, the art of living must be sculpted and created as a way of life.

The art of living can be practiced by the simplest act of following ordinary impulses, to trust in the moment by moment assistance of any inner urging that holds the key to the fulfillment of my destiny. Our society warns against the following of impulses in general because they go against a logical and rational reason for action. And as children, most of us are taught to tame our impulsive side, because it is unsafe, even dangerous.

But in order to practice the art of living, I was led to see that my spontaneous urging were therapeutic steps furthering my expression towards creativity, whether to change my place of residence, to dance all night, to eat a particular food, to write down an idea, or simply to pause a moment to appreciate the new day. The art of living meant regarding the self and all people as intrinsically good. I had to learn to ignore the media messages that emphasized the weakness of the physical body, and of the violent nature of human beings. I wanted to free my mind from these hampering beliefs that created a fearful state and hindered trust of my own abilities.

I knew my gifts to the world would flower naturally using this method. I would not pursue my abilities hoping to gain fame or wealth, but would do so for the enjoyment and fulfillment of my selfhood. The simple acceptance of my place in the universe would generate a climate for realized potential without comparing talents to societal norms or to those in my immediate world. Suspicion of our impulses leads to a deep mistrust of life and the need to justify experience by rigid rules and an over compensation for any one particular talent as the excuse for individual existence.

Animals have perfect faith of their place in the universe, as do infants and children. Faith is the foundation of all of nature, for doesn't summer follow the rebirth of spring and the rising sun give hope of a new day? These cycles are given to us and accepted without question.

In this way, the urge for action rises out of the inner workings of faith. Action gives momentum and direction to our goals, leading to an overall comprehension concerning the whole of life.

Nevertheless, most people view impulses as dangerous, leading surely to destructive tendencies inherent in the evil core of human nature. Some people think they have a good spiritual inner self whom can be looked to for guidance, but the familiar, focused self is flawed, therefore to be mistrusted. The trick to gaining self knowledge is to get rid of these unnecessary divisions, and accept all aspects of the self, thus promoting the experience of self unity.

Our inner selves are not elusive or abstract but exist within every cell of our body, just as God exists within all creation. Our inner selves contact us by our own passing thoughts or by connecting with strangers in an elevator.

I wanted to acknowledge the freedom of each impulse as a symbol for the inner movement towards the ideal of what I wanted life to be. These urges are the life-giving impetus towards personal growth. As I learned to recognize and follow through with my own impulses, they no longer seemed contrary to my goals and aspirations.

Private actions reverberate outwardly to affect the action of the world in a circuit of activity originating on inner levels. By formulating a picture of the human species as one of good intent, and by trusting the forward movement of one's personal life as taking care of itself, it is not necessary to understand how the universe works other than to have the simple yet profound faith that it does.

As I prepared to go into nursing, I placed more value on my own excellent health. I hoped to teach others the knack of staying well, themselves. This presupposed a deep inner knowledge of myself which I could encourage in others for the purpose of strengthening and reinforcing spiritual knowledge. I envisioned that my specialty in medicine was to teach the dynamics between vitality and physical well-being for ideally, not only does the body have the capacity for excellent health, it also has the capacity to maintain a high level of physical achievement.

We can look to our greatest athletes as proof of this. The ordained Buddhist Monks from the Shaolin Temple in China, proficient in Kung-Fu, also point to inner poise and power manifesting in great physical achievement originating from spiritual strength.

One cannot help others by taking on their troubles, nor can the world be saved by carrying burdens as a sign of caring. It is far more practical to concentrate upon the beneficial aspects of the culture and to observe the accomplishments of people, rather than making mental lists of their deficiencies and lacks, thus eliminating effective action.

The idea is not to ignore the dire circumstances of the world, but to acknowledge one's own strength and creativity, and from that viewpoint, look at those areas in need of constructive help.

I felt it was important to enlarge upon feelings of well-being and spontaneity and to encourage the feelings and activities that bring them about. Unfortunate life situations should have no power over us if we realize that events do not exist by themselves; they exist first in the mind. If every person changed her attitude to encompass all that is wonderful about life, tomorrow, the world will change for the better. Empowering new laws would follow.

The ideal is to join with every human being, all living creatures, the sun, earth, wind and flower. Prayer connects us to all things in the universe. This is why it works so well to bring healing.

Another ancient art that is powerfully helpful is to tune into the message of our dreams. This requires an acknowledgment that beneath the world we know, there is another. Adjacent to our familiar focus there are other realities that are just as legitimate. We can draw from these worlds to heal our lives.

Long term illnesses have often resolved suddenly through a dream or dream series. Dreams often allow for the prevention of a chronic condition without our having any conscious awareness of how this happens.

I had a vision for my calling as a nurse. I wanted to be the kind of person who could stimulate my patients to pursue personal potential in a strictly unique style, to pursue and develop awareness as a prerequisite to peace of mind. The official, accepted view of the world no longer applied, then and now, as new suppositions of the will are built upon and encouraged to evolve, bringing a new base and foundation upon which to formulate individual and cultural action, as a manifestation of life-as art form.

Medicine as an art form rests on these principles: a spontaneous and life giving approach, an evaluation of exteriorly manifested conditions as a reflection of attitudes and beliefs, and the act of remaining flexible and playful in one's approach to life. The choice is a personal one. But once the journey has begun, the adventure becomes a colorful kaleidoscope of unpredictable action; the art-form never finished, always giving to new creation.

Chapter Twenty-Three: Mystics in the Workplace

Once the calling has reverberated in every cell of the nurse's body, she is ready to make a difference in the world. The image of Jesus in the market place over turning tables and expressing his feelings against a materialistic world gone mad yet all the while maintaining his equilibrium and center of peace, is an example of a mystic in the world who has not gone to reside permanently on the mountaintop.

A nurse must not abandon her calling. She must confront the barriers that obscure the initial feeling of destiny regarding her deeply held conviction of what nursing originally meant to her.

My twelfth year serving the York City and County community as Nurse Practitioner was harder since the move to the inner city. Dr. O., the latest slash and burn Ob/Gyn rookie resident, reduced two women to tears a few days ago. These women were new employees. The computer displayed an ever lengthening list of patients who needed to be brought back to the exam rooms for evaluation, then to be seen by a doctor or Nurse Practitioner. This happens all the time. The patients always are seen. But this time, Dr. O. screamed at the new nurses, blamed them for the patient back up, paced back and forth like a drill sergeant and consequently the nurses froze and were unable to perform with optimal flow.

She said, "Nurses should not question a doctor's order. Her job is just to carry it out."

One of the nurses targeted by the wrath of Dr. O. had a stroke while at work, today. She was transported by ambulance to the hospital emergency room.

Our workplace lacks a basic component that if allowed to thrive, would save it from self destruction: Emotional Intelligence.

Everyone must take responsibility for any and all failings of the workplace organization. Also, any great deeds and positive accomplishments are the result of the team as a whole whose energy allowed the momentum to move in the direction of the great achievement. The trick is to stop projecting our power, both negative and positive, outside of ourselves and then giving credit or blame to other people.

The most insightful guide for creating work place excellence is the Emotional Intelligent model, as made popular by Daniel Goldman, a former behavioral scientific writer for the New York Times.

Emotional intelligence refers to *THE CAPACITY FOR RECOGNIZING OUR OWN FEELINGS AND THOSE OF OTHERS, FOR MOTIVATING OURSELVES, AND FOR MANAGING EMOTIONS WELL IN OURSELVES AND IN OUR RELATIONSHIPS*, Dr. Goldman writes. It describes abilities distinct from, but complementary to, academic intelligence, the purely cognitive capabilities measured by IQ. Many people who are book smart but lack emotional intelligence end up working for people who have lower IQs than they do but excel in emotional intelligent skills.

Emotional intelligence must begin with the leadership of the organization. Studies show that if an employee respects and likes her boss, she will stay and work hard at her respective job, and overall staff retention results.

The boss must help to create group flow and synergy in pursuing collective goals. She must model team qualities like respect, helpfulness and cooperation. She must draw all members into active and enthusiastic participation. She must build team spirit and commitment.

She must not take credit but share credit for team accomplishments.

And until this becomes a reality, small pockets of enlightened potential shine on and off, like tinkerbells in the workplace, pleading for the opportunity to shine consistently in a supportive environment.

In order for emotional intelligence to take hold in any organization, intensive training must take place, first of all with supervisors who have made the commitment to develop emotional intelligence as a way of life.

These supervisors develop:
1) self awareness, that is, knowing how she feels at all times
2) self regulation, that is, managing one's internal states and impulses
3) motivation, that is, the ability to guide or facilitate the reaching of goals despite obstacles or setbacks.

Leaders must also develop:
4) empathy, that is, awareness of other people's feelings, needs and concerns.

The New York Times had a special daily

column dedicated to those who were lost in the World Trade Center terrorist attack, written since 9/11/01, entitled PORTRAITS IN GRIEF. The people who were commemorated there exemplify all the emotional intelligent qualities that are necessary for companies and businesses to succeed, originating with the people who comprise them.

They all had in common a wide range of interests and activities, an immense influence of people who loved them, an abundant sense of humor, the ability to laugh and make others laugh with them. I believe *PORTRAITS IN GRIEF* should be required reading for those who wish to study and emulate models of emotional intelligence.

A tragic flaw of any organization is if the leadership refuses to recognize the problems within an already crumbling structure. Leadership must take responsibility for the good and the bad before full potential can be realized, and the talent and creativity of the staff can flourish.

PART THREE: Staying Awake: Creating the Compassionate Organization

An angel is watching the nurses, the doctors, the secretaries and all the patients go about a few minutes of a typical workday from a treetop near the Community Health Center. She asks herself, "What can I do to make them happy?"

She further ponders, "Would it be morally ethical for me to wave my wand and automatically give happiness when the recipient of my gift may not even want to be happy? They don't seem to know the first thing about happiness. The nurses don't stand up for themselves, the staff seems to think that happiness awaits them at the end of a work day, the resident doctors haven't had enough life experience to know what true happiness is.

"My greatest gift to them is to allow these people to discover for themselves the true meaning of happiness."

She does wave her wand, then. A presence is felt by those who are open to other worldly messages. They suddenly feel a sense of balance and then begin to work in the world with a innate feeling of self and selflessness.

Chapter Twenty-Four: From Basement to Boundary

The move to the building of windows was completed in the year 2000. Some of my patients feel they were raised in the clinic cave that we left behind.

They tell me they loved that old place with vomit green painted walls, staff literally tripping over one another, and posters lining the hallway filled to capacity with baby pictures of our patients. Now those pictures are in my new office, jammed behind a trash can, threatening to turn yellow with age if we do not soon preserve them.

The windows span around the entire building. Only the rooms that are centrally located do not have a window with a city scape. My desk faced out on the parking lot where our patients parked. I saw them come and go. I could sense their mood, whether they were ill or well. The sky revealed an occasional crow flying near my level of observation. Across the way on a rooftop flew an American flag, so placed since the 9/11/01 terrorist attack.

I never thought I'd miss the crowded office we all shared when we were on top of one another in the basement clinic. I don't miss the harshness of fluorescence. But the spontaneous outbursts and stress releasing comments were great fun, in retrospect. I loved it when we put on a classical musical C-D and said we were in our inner sanctuary. Or at the end of the day when we could chat about a vacation just taken or the anticipation of a trip or educational experience and what we hoped would happen or be learned.

One of my former office mates brought me into her office the other evening as the sun was setting. She said her window offered the best view of the sunset in the entire building, and she was right. I knew which window to see the rising of the moon. I knew where the best vantage point was for the first day of the new moon, and as the moon mellowed and grew larger, which window to view her luminous beauty. As autumn and winter merged, the clouds gave unique displays of the ever changing qualities of each day, one day never the same as any other.

When I used to invite someone to view a cloud with me, and she said, "I'm too busy for that," and hurried on with grim determination, I knew that pockets of the workplace have fallen from a state of grace.

I saw patients every Wednesday afternoon with the help of a nurse. I had a big room lined with windows all to myself. The leaves had fallen off the trees. The large expanse of street overlooking old architectural structures of the town with five pigeons roosting on an old chimney structure, looking at me as I suddenly saw them, had a soothing effect on my psyche.

Only then do I know that all the comradery in small windowless spaces with stark fluorescence burning eyes and energy can not compete with this new experience of solitary patient care with the sudden realization that a long line of ancestral pigeons were giving me strength to seize each day with a thankful and joyful presence.

Chapter Twenty-Five: Doing Time on Planet Earth

I am thinking about what has brought joy to the great thinkers and spiritual giants who have lived and died on this planet. Usually, it is the simple acts that inspire. In reality, there is no difference between a prisoner behind bars, a monk in a monastery, a drunk in a tavern, or a person who arises every day to set about the task of working in the world. Freedom, after all, is in the mind. Every one of us can strive to be free.

I write these words, walking the dogs on a trail that winds along the Mill Stream in late autumn. We have just encountered a yellow lab. The dogs danced and played together for a time, then parted ways, the dogs grinning even wider than before, if that is possible. We can learn so much about love from the animals in our lives and in medicine especially, if we allow them to enter the front door of the sterile institution, to sooth troubled souls, and bring to the anxious a moment of peace.

But we are just doing time as we watch the time clock, and do not sense the opportunities for greater understanding inherent in each moment. If we do not reach out in a spirit of helping or for connection, we have missed the greater meaning of what life is all about. We are just doing time if we think we have to be right, that there is only one point of view, that there is only one religion, if we do not sense the poetic potential in each experience.

The only limits are the ones we place upon our lives.

Chapter Twenty-Six: The Angels are With Us

There was a world wide meditation at 11:11 a.m. on 11/11/01, exactly two months after the terrorist attack. We were to collectively visualize a band of angels circling Afghanistan, beaming peaceful waves to all people in that country and in the world. We sat with our wet dogs on the trail next to the Mill Stream, and sent out our thoughts of peace to the angels there and everywhere. It has been the warmest autumn in memory, with perfect blue skies and brilliantly colored leaves, now fallen to reveal the natural contours of the brown earth.

I want to draw on that angelic energy in all activities. The dogs are themselves angels. It is easy to feel love, be loved and to give love while in their presence.

Now that the weather has cooled down and the days are shorter, I take the dogs to work every Thursday, and park in full view of the pediatric exam room windows that look down on the boys as they peer out watching squirrels or look up at us when we tap on the windows to get their attention.

I take a child to the window to look at the dogs

immediately after an immunization. They stop crying and point at the majestic beauty of the now seven month Golden Retriever, Ulysses, who is in the company of his wise five year companion, Mukunda, who sits on the floor out of view. We take long walks at lunch time and before we go home at night, meeting my patients along the way who admire and smile at the two playful beasts.

The days I bring the dogs creates a unified feeling to the pediatric staff, and all others who see them. My own mood is greatly improved. I feel more like laughing, making jokes, just because I know the boys are with me.

An angel on each shoulder, furry ones with long wavy coats.

Chapter Twenty-Seven: Angels of Mercy

Let the angels go before us, clearing the path of all obstacles, including the negative thought fields of fear, anxiety, lack of forgiveness and resentment.

Imagine the beautiful luminescent wings of beauty clearing out the old, and bringing love and protection in its place.

This is what we can do in our work-become one with our angels, have a close feeling of companionship with them, feel their eternal loving presence, and welcome them again and again into our hearts.

Ask them to help in emergency situations. Ask them to help in times of suffering, that they may leave a glimmer of joy for us to use for the transformation of self, leading to the One Self.

Ask them to help us remember their Love and their help which is always available. For in our forgetting, we feel alone, we feel vulnerable, and we lose the strength that we need to co-create with our unseen helpers and friends.

Nurses are called angels of mercy. We are often told: "You were my angel and I thank you."

Yes this is true but the only way we can sustain angelic heights in our work is to always ask the angels to be with us–now and forever. Om Peace Amen.

Chapter Twenty-Eight: The End of Human Dominion

The main premise of scientific, religious and every day inquiry centers around the understanding that humans are superior to all other life forms. And indeed, that humans are the only conscious entities in the universe.

Because of this premise, a wide range of heartless experiments are performed on primates and all other animals, to supposedly further man's understanding of herself, of the human brain, of disease states, and in the development of cosmetics and pharmaceutical medicines, to name just a few examples.

The Harlow rhesus monkey experiments are the one great example of pure idiocy that insults without enlightenment. The experiment describes so well our laise-faire attitude towards the suffering of these poor creatures.

The Harlow rhesus monkey experiment is well known to anyone who has taken a Psychology 101 class. It describes the removal of rhesus monkey babies from their mother, caging each one of them separately in a windowless environment, depriving them of touch or stimulation of any kind: in short, proving that a human child must have love and touch in order to thrive, never thinking that these deprivations would create a seething enraged monster who would kill anything in her path if left to go free.

I personally met the offspring of the Harlow monkeys at a psychology lab at a local ivy league college in my home town. I learned from a psychologist friend of mine who taught at the college that these monkeys were housed in the basement of his workplace. I begged him to introduce them to me.

He gave me a few instructions before he took me to their prison. "Don't make eye contact with them, whatever you do," he said. I decided that eye contact would most assuredly teach me what I needed to learn from them.

It took about five minutes to get to the Primate Research Lab in the building. It was well hidden. My friend was taking a risk by bringing me there.

Perhaps he would lose his job if we were discovered.

Long before entering, I could smell the stench of feces and urine. My friend put on a dim light in an already darkened room. My first vivid observation was a red beam of light emanating from the eyes of the six monkeys who resided there. Anger red. Their primate hands gripped the bars and shook the walls with their fury. One or two jumped up and down. They threw excrement at us. They were well secured but I feared for my life if even one of them broke out.

Do we really need to prove the obvious: that any animal deprived of love will be violent and imbalanced? Do we need to conduct research on the chimpanzee brain to further our understanding of motivational states, such as hunger, thirst or emotion? People who glibly conduct these experiments have lost their common sense. We are as much at fault as they are because we allow it to happen.

In his landmark book, *RATTLING THE CAGE*, Steven M. Wise has written eloquently for the equal rights of chimpanzees and bonobos, and hence, all other animals.

I was horrified to read about the ASL (American Sign Language) adept chimpanzee named Lucy who was the offspring of a carnival couple and was raised for twelve years by psychologists. They completely socialized her, then after many years, could no longer care for her. She was flown to a chimpanzee rehabilitation center in Senegal. She was then flown to Gambia after a difficult adjustment period. Poachers shot and skinned her. Her feet and hands were severed and sold as trophies.

A language using chimpanzee has never been exempt from the deadly biomedical research and testing where she is subjected to invasive brain studies that kill her. Yet why exempt some monkeys from research and not others? Obviously they must all be exempt. And they must all be protected in the wild immediately or soon they will be extinct.

By giving primates entitlement to fundamental legal rights, we will go a long way to stop the abuse of these creatures. We need a deus ex machina experience to reverse the momentum towards extinction of their species.

The whole idea of human dominion must be eradicated before we can hope to have a society of respect and civility. My dogs may not know American Sign Language but they understand everything that I say, at least on an emotional level. My dogs unconditionally love me more than anyone else ever has. They do this automatically and spontaneously. It is time that humans learn lessons of love from all other creatures not by imprisoning them, but by allowing the free expression of love to flow through all things, and letting go in the process.

Only then will we know what true equality is.

Chapter Twenty-Nine: Relinquishing the Ego

Our Community Health Care Center serves an inner city poor population. Some have made the adjustment to this setting more smoothly than others. But our patients pose special challenges to us that others working in more affluent settings may not have to face, or face less often. We see more chronic illness, hunger, violence, alcoholism, domestic abuse, addiction, depression, anxiety, hopelessness and potential for suicide, sometimes all in the same person, than in other health care settings. Our time to deal with these problems is getting more crunched into twenty, more often ten minute time slots. We may feel that our ability to truly make a difference is compromised by these limitations in time.

Furthermore, gangs of children began to target our facility and harass people with new cars. The other evening eight children, ages 7-12, silently entered the office of one of the employees, took her pocket book with keys to her car and to the building. They immediately found her car with the automatic button on her key chain, and were about to steal it. The office worker saw her car lights blinking off and on from her office window, called 911, grabbed the male cleaning person and went outside to confront the children.

Evidently, the confrontation was carried out in a spirit of anger. The police did eventually come, but not fast enough. Three kids were apprehended, but five others made off with the pocketbook and keys, wallet, and credit cards, all intact.

The staff was never gathered together and appraised of the situation. We were never told, as a group, what had actually taken place. During the course of the following day, when visiting the zerox machine or getting a cup of tea, a person would excitedly offer new shreds of information, that may or may not have been true, to piece together the puzzles of the story.

I remembered playing ball in the parking lot with a group of children and my dog not too many months before. I remembered thinking: the children see us as separate entities, people who are removed from their lives up there in our new medical arts building. I've played with the children a few times since, with the dog they already knew and the new puppy, Ulysses. They seem to need some attention from us, I remembered thinking, and do not need to see us escorted to our cars by security officers, because we are afraid of them.

For our community health center to survive, we need to focus on our vision of idealism in providing health care to the poor and under served. In the strength of our mission, we will attract talented health care workers and personnel who identify with the mission and with the obvious need of our services to the community we serve. We all need to be actively involved in creating a mission statement that reflects our collective and unique talents in making the mission a reality.

When people believe in the work that they are doing, an atmosphere of cooperation naturally develops. The us vs. them mentality vanishes. A sense of selflessness, detachment and joy in the pure act of carrying out tasks in the moment develops when a loving link is made to our patients, coworkers, and the person outside, crossing the street.

Chapter Thirty: Tears and Healing

I cried today, and felt immediately better. I wrote a letter saying I was sorry to someone I may have hurt. I took my dogs for a walk in the rain and watched them play in the mud, knowing that water would ultimately wash it away.

Men find it difficult to cry in American culture. It is a taboo. But when a woman cries, a great deal of concern also arises. What could be wrong? What needs to be done to comfort her?

The chemical composition of tears of joy and tears of sorrow are different. Yet to shed tears of any kind needs to be actively developed if life is to become a fully evolving reflection of who a person really is.

We have all been taught not to cry with our patients. It is considered a weakness. We are taught in nursing school not to touch our patients. The patient may take it the wrong way.

Once a person has been given the foundations of medicine and nursing in school, then goes forth to work with patients for many years, at some point the heart and intuition start playing a more prominent role in critical decision making regarding a patient's plan of care. We can feel when something is not right, when a person is telling the truth, or not. We develop an innate commonsense ability as to how to proceed in any given scenario with our patients. Our patients, in turn, know if we are not being authentic, and may or may not tell us about it, depending on the depth of our relationship, or how long it has been developing.

I know one thing: tears wash the spirit clean. An injustice is served when antidepressants are prescribed at the first sign of a tear. A good cry and a hearty laugh are not diametrically opposed. In fact, the body, mind and soul is cleansed of the toxic buildup of stress with both laughing and crying. By welcoming the free flow of emotions in ourselves and others, we feel better. We are in tune. And major disease may have been thwarted.

Chapter Thirty-One: Listening

The receptive mind is openly conscious and awake, listening for messages from the inner world of thought and dreams, and to the outer world often swirling with distraction and stimulation. Learning to balance these two worlds is the secret leading to peace of mind and happiness.

The art of writing, music, painting, prayer, war, peace, medicine and nursing requires a mind that listens fully in the present moment. I write these words, and I listen. I hear a gentle rain, occasional far-away thunder, the breathing of two sleeping dogs lying by my side. I smell the freshness of the first rain in weeks and can taste the fullness of moisture in the air. This small but fully dimensioned experience is there for anyone willing to slow down and feel the pulsation of heaven and earth in the space of a single second.

Hearing the rain on the roof, smelling the 60 degree breezes, places my consciousness in between worlds. I think of all the times I have listened or not listened to our patients. Not listening produces disastrous results that only lack of connection produces. Listening lies down a rock bed of strength that nothing ever destroys.

The art of listening requires a presence of attention without crossed legs, no hand upon the door, no desk between you and your patient. It requires a balance between allowing all to be said and remembering pieces of what was said to be brought up again for clarity of understanding, such as any dangerous red flags that need to be further explored, like homicidal or suicidal ideation. We need to elaborate upon the positives such as love of family, children, other people and of the self. Listening well, allowing all to flow, is a kind of meditation. Getting out of the way, keeping your agenda as a blank slate, allows trust to develop naturally.

And when many patients need to be seen over the course of the day, listening becomes a form of self-preservation and regeneration.

Experiencing all people who come to us for care as brothers and sisters allows full attention to be channeled for the larger good of all concerned in a dance of daily creation.

Chapter Thirty-Two: Practicing Forgiveness

My patients who have been raped, violently attacked, or molested as children have life long challenges forgiving their perpetrators. Forgiveness often is not seen as an option. Yet hanging on to hurt for years causes a type of mental illness borne from hate that creates a seething round and round relentless inner voice that urges for revenge.

The choice to forgive is a choice to transform, to begin again in a spirit of connection with all of life. Choosing not to forgive continues a cycle of fragmentation, of cycles repeated again and again, where no growth can ever occur. To choose again implies putting one's faith with the angels and with God.

As an old Rabbi once said, "Love your neighbor as if he IS yourself." In that state of mind, communion with the person who committed the wrong occurs and the steps towards forgiveness have begun.

Forgiveness, then, is a moment of complete release, when suddenly all past confusion is made clear. Heart to heart connections make all that happened in the hurtful past a memory made light by revelation. Only if the pain of the past has honestly been felt, layer by layer, can true forgiveness occur. Trying to escape from the pain will not make it possible to forgive.

Forgiveness releases negativity and leaves a void, an emptiness allowing for hope of a new beginning, like a re-birth, the start of a whole new life that feels light, loving and innocent.

As an exercise in detachment, I tell my patients to imagine Planet Earth revolving in space, visualized from a great distance. From this perspective, all of our personal and global troubles fade, replaced by a feeling of unity. This vision may occur after one or several visualizations, but at some point, a momentary sense of clarity, a sense of Eureka! And an understanding that all is not as it originally seemed settles into your consciousness.

The pain is in the fragmentation, and is not part of the larger perspective. With this new realization, the work of forgiveness makes sense, and the pure practical beauty of it makes the work worth doing.

Forgiveness becomes the only true option.

Chapter Thirty-Three: Balance and Protection

In order to be effective in her work, a nurse needs to be centered, balanced and aligned with her highest source of guidance. Daily meditation and an attitude of prayer at every moment is a prerequisite for achieving an experience of peace in work and all other areas of her life.

To the young men and women who wish to enter the nursing profession now but feel conflicted about doing so, a few soulful questions need to be pondered.

Do you feel a calling to serve?

Can you sustain this vision throughout a grueling educational experience and resurrect it daily in the years of daily work?

Are you willing to be a patient advocate no matter what?

Are you ready to be an advocate for nursing as a profession which now appears poised for extinction?

Can you find the balance within yourself to give selflessly and at the same time, save for yourself moments of solitude, times for exercise and good nutrition that uphold the determination to persevere, often in the face of great human misery and also resilience, as exemplified in the lives of our patients?

Finding the balance within is a form of protection. No one will take care of us if we do not first take care of ourselves. Learning to collectively say "No" to mandatory overtime, to the doctors who mistreat us, to the insurance companies whose CEOs see more money in a year than our patients will ever see, is an exercise in creating a strong inner reserve that will serve our profession in the coming years.

Chapter Thirty-Four: Ageism

"Life begins at 50."

"Youth is wasted on the young."

These are truisms that our society largely ignores. Yet there is a growing movement of people who wish to grow old consciously, who see the last stage of life as a period of growth and transformation, not as a time when nursing home care is inevitable, senility takes over, incontinence and bedsores are the only reality.

Women in our society are living longer and adjusting more holistically to aging than our male counterparts. Conversely, women over 65 are the fastest growing demographic who end up the poorest of the poor in the American community. This is due in part to the elimination of social security for those who did not earn wages during the child rearing years and then, because of divorce, do not receive that entitlement after age 65. I am surprised this law found its way into public policy in an age when women imagine themselves to be so much more liberated than say, women under the former Taliban rule.

Growing old is perceived as a problem in American culture. Scientific studies and the media concentrate on deteriorating brain cells, on slower neurologic response, on the rising cancer and chronic illness rates. Furthermore, women are viewed as wives, mothers, and sex objects to men and servers to the needs of husbands, children and the home. But women are changing these roles as they age, taking on professional and entrepreneurial careers, feeling in control of their personal and collective destinies and are aging more gracefully than men.

Women are in the position to take these negative stereotypes about aging and change them forever. The same women who lived through the 1960's and participated in the Vietnam anti-war movement and the sexual revolution will all be aging at the same time and at a record number. We can take that flame from our idealized youthful years and reignite that energy to change the world forever. When the worn out views about aging are replaced with an energetic embracing of who we are meant to be, conscious growth will evolve and the new millennium will truly be the New Age.

Chapter Thirty-Five: Suffering

Suffering is one of the truths of our physical existence. One must go through it in order to get to the other side where a greater meaning awaits. Avoidance of suffering creates more of the same as well as different kinds of torment, all layered tightly, waiting for release.

Falling into patterns of blame and revenge; holding onto past hurts and refusing to forgive perpetrates more inner pain, often manifesting as societal threat in the form of murder, suicide, addiction and all manner of violent acts.

A person often imagines she is alone in her great sadness. But by visualizing that all others in the world have pain like hers or greater, it is possible to fill the heart with compassion for them. She prays to whomever she believes in, and asks that her suffering helps to alleviate theirs. If she again and again dedicates her pain to the alleviation of their pain, she will discover within herself a new source of strength and will feel that her suffering is not being wasted. It now has a wonderful new meaning.

It is said that the great Tibetan masters bring

the pain of the world into themselves with every in breath, and release healing and love to the world with every out breath, every moment of their enlightened lives. Their love and compassion is so boundless, the teachings say, that at the moment of their death they are reborn immediately into the Buddha realm.

We do not have to be enlightened masters to do this simple but moving exercise. But to do it may take us further along the path of our journey than we ever imagined we could go.

Chapter Thirty-Six: Compassion

At the heart of all human motivation is the urge, the pull towards happiness. But when our actions lack compassion and bring frustration and discomfort not only to ourselves but to everyone around us, only unhappiness results. The search for happiness feels elusive, at best. It seems that all our actions and purposes lead directly away from the harmony that we seek.

In reality, happiness can not be found in material pursuits, nor does control over others bring an experience of fulfillment. Every single negative thing ever thought or done arises from our identification with a false self who sees with loveless perception. This perception makes unconditional love and the compassion that arises out of that a dim promise.

Yet it is the daily practice of compassion that washes away all the anguish of confused and hurtful relationships and the inner turmoil we feel within ourselves. The opportunities for practice abound in every day life. As nurses, all of our patients suffer and we can guide healing energy directly to them with every breath. The suffering brought about during and after the 9/11/01 terrorist attack opened endless channels to direct the energy.

This energy is made of pure love and is waiting to be used for the greater good. We do not need to recoil in fear at all the suffering in the world, but open ourselves to it and use it as a conduit in which to pour all of our love.

We pray that we benefit all who contact us and that their suffering may be transformed by the energy we help direct their way.

Chapter Thirty-Seven: Attraction/Aversion

I once heard a lecture given by Ram Dass in which he said that the sum total of a person's karma is reflected in what that person feels attraction for or aversion against. And to wipe out karma, or endless reincarnational cycles, all one needs to do is to stop having strong likes and dislikes towards people, experiences and the circumstances we resist in our lives.

We have the choice of how to experience our own daily stories as they enfold. The simple idea of seeing all of physical life as a school room, a learning experience, and perceive all the players as ourselves, is a first step. Then, as Ram Dass says, remembering to love and serve everyone and to remember God, are the instructions from the classroom. These are the only acts worth doing and doing well. Or if not always done well, to forgive and love yourself for trying and to begin once again.

I must move beyond my role as nurse if I want my patients to be who they really are in my presence. The essence of service is to experience less and less the feeling that those we serve are apart from ourselves. Since we are all one, then my interactions must arise apart from the separation that typifies most day to day contact.

Our desires dictate our experience. If a pick pocket meets a saint, all she sees are her pockets. This is what we must learn to move away from and see the soul of those we meet, the essence of that which never dies. It is by moving out of the duality, the me verses you mentality, that leads to true liberation.

Chapter Thirty-Eight: Transformation of the Self

I went to a ten day workshop several years ago specifically designed to transform me forever. The vehicle for doing this was through the energy fields of the body, where we learned to experience and heal them. In order to be healed, we had to honestly want to change our lives, sometimes in dramatic ways. We had to decide to think with the heart and let the intellect gently out the door. We learned to be kind to ourselves, some for the first time. We learned about our own natural rhythms for rest and action, and learned to distinguish between them.

In order to sustain this feeling of renewal after the ten days were over, a daily practice of meditation was necessary so as to build upon the transformative process. A daily conscious discipline helps to reduce the power of negative emotions such as anger or hatred, and naturally encourages the antidote: love and compassion. Meditation plugs us into that nonphysical realm where rebirth and regeneration are enfolding all the time. A daily sustained effort is required to cultivate positive aspects within ourselves.

Mindfulness, or living in the present moment, is a practice well suited for the times spent between sitting meditation. Mindfulness is practiced with every breath, every step, every bite of food, while listening to words spoken or unspoken. The rhythm of every in and out breath is the focus of this discipline. The simple act of breathing takes on whole worlds of depth and meaning.

And it is through these practices that transformation of self evolves.

Chapter Thirty-Nine: Transforming the Medical System

The answer is clear: the medical system can not be transformed unless those working within that system transform themselves.

Transformation of self reverberates outward to lift the consciousness of the whole. This happens first in small pockets, builds momentum and overtakes the entire medical system in America!

As Saint Francis of Assisi once said: "Sanctify yourself And you sanctify society."

Let's do it!

Chapter Forty: Healing and the Natural World

There are little people who live at the base of Mount Shasta near Redding, California. Not exactly little people, but small gnomes, with hats. Some of them use sticks to maneuver in and around the rocks. They occupy another realm apart from the one we normally occupy, but some people have seen them. I know, because I've seen them, too.

I was with friends and we planned to hike all the way to the top of the 10,000 foot mountain. Yet from the walk's beginning, I kept catching fleeting movements out of the corner of my eye. These movements became more persistent, and if I was ignoring what I thought I was seeing, I could no longer. Then I began seeing them straight on, populated most densely around the many boulders, in great numbers. They were not paying any attention to me, but were involved with tasks that appeared to involve great concentration. I stopped and marveled at suddenly finding myself in another dimension. It propelled my consciousness in what felt like a dream. I wanted to lie down and go to sleep, like Rip Van Winkle.

My friends were impatient with me for slowing down. One of them came back to see if anything was wrong. I assumed she could see them, too. She could not.

Great waves of doubt overcame my mind as we went further up the mountain to set up camp for the night. I felt I must have imagined these little people. But I was sure I saw them. Or did I? Was it simply a case of altitude sickness? If true, once I acclimated for the next three days, the length of our intended stay, I was sure I would not see them on the way down. In fact, I was sure I would not.

The next three days we explored the mountain, hiked to the top, experienced the world on top of a 10,000 foot peak. We heard rock avalanches in the depth of night, and became one with the mountain and each other. I forgot about the little people.

On the way down, in the foothills once again, I felt and saw the presence of the little people moving about the rocks, fulfilling tasks I could not fathom. This time I was sure, clear headed from several days of hard and exhilarating exercise and full sun upon my body, that they existed, as surely as I or anyone else exist.

What else do we miss because of our

judgements, preconceptions and speed of thought?

I later discovered a metaphysical bookstore in the town of Mount Shasta. Several books about the little people of that mountain were prominently displayed. The proprietors of the bookstore told me that the legend of the little people of Mount Shasta is well known among the townspeople. The American Indians of the area co-mingled with them. Perhaps help was elicited from their prestigious ability to work and carry out tasks.

Perhaps all of that concentrated energy helped avert volcanic disaster.

They are there, to this day. I must go again to feel that determination, that dream-like feeling of slipping into another world, the healing that comes from touching other universes. In truth, I will step out my door tonight and feel the presence of tree spirits, and river gnomes. The yelp of the red-fox will electrify. The hoot of the night owl will quiet tension. It is all a matter of slowing down, learning to live between the worlds that occupy many dimensions.

This is what nature teaches us. This is how nature heals.

Chapter Forty-One: Life is But a Dream

My father died a year ago, today. He was 88, his body had failed him and it was time to move on to the next classroom of learning. He died in the Emergency Room of the hometown hospital. A nun was with him. She put her hand on his chest and said, "Does your chest hurt, Franklin?" And he said, "Only when you lean on it." They both smiled at his joke, and off he went.

We had a memorial service for him on his birthday, six months later. While the minister and good friend read a poem my father had written, several butterflies lightly touched her head. A hush fell on the crowd who had gathered to honor him. I was wearing a shimmering butterfly shirt that seemed to be made of tiny jewels. My father approved of our efforts to memorialize him.

And now, as time has taken on a speed that no one can halt, I look back over the past 50 years of my own life. There are no guarantees as to how much more time is left. To live as long as my father or his sister, who is ninety- two, to love every moment along the way, to feel the warmth of benevolence surrounding the planet, and most importantly, to close every door with grace and humility are wonderful acts of faith achieved with a simple heart.

The river outside my window refracts light from the dawn. The light grows brighter with each magnificent microsecond, and I know that we will carry it off. Nursing will weather the storms of restlessness and we will come home again to be the profession exemplified by individual acts of great service and love for every patient. Nothing can stop us now. But we must collectively take a stand for who we are and how much more we can achieve.

The promise of the predawn pale rosy glow ignites my heart and makes it possible to find the essence and integrity of what it means to create the true energy of nursing.

Chapter Forty-Two: The New Years Baby

Every day is a new opportunity to begin again especially for those who choose to make amends for past hurts, or who choose love over fear regarding experience or lessons learned from other people.

Sometimes it is a brand new day entirely and that day comes once in a lifetime-at the moment of one's birth. If that day merges within the first few moments of the New Year, as everyone on the planet renews an inner pledge to be better people, to love and forgive more fully, to live healthier and with more appreciation–even if this desired renewal is unconscious in the hearts of many: The heavens meet the earth to herald in a new life.

Every birth is a monumental vibrational event, but when coinciding with that first beginning of a new year, the heart of the entire community rejoices.

So it was New Year's Day 2005 @ 0008 or 1208 a.m. when the first baby of the year in our particular county was born. I participated in the birth. My role was to coach the patient and to receive the baby whenever she decided to show up. My shift began at 2300 0r 1100 p.m. and the patient, Roxanne, had been pushing exactly one hour by the time I got there. My friend and colleague, Paula, was also working with me. Her main responsibility was to stabilize Roxanne after the birth.

The room was ninety degrees even though the air conditioning was turned up as far as it would go. The family standing around the bed has a glistening quality to their skin. They fanned one another as well as Roxanne, who was saturated. Roxanne's husband and sisters placed cool rags on her forehead. It felt like a sweat lodge in that room.

Roxanne got into the rhythm of pushing and was doing beautifully. With every push, we could see more and more of the baby's head. The feeling of expectancy was joyous. The angelic realm was filling up all of the empty spaces everywhere in the room.

Then at 0008 the body of the baby made its first grand entrance. But she was limp and her eyes were startled like those of a deer in the headlights of a car. We stimulated her, gave her oxygen, and she still appeared to be almost lifeless, although her heart rate was perfectly normal. She also was breathing normally.

Suddenly, a look of surprise registered on her tiny face: a look of OH! I am supposed to be here, now! It was if the soul had been out and about and then decided to make her grand re-entry.

In retrospect, I decided that birth and death have one major difference. At birth, the soul enters the body, and at death, the soul exits the body. The angels are there at both events. The trick is to honor their sacred presence.

As the baby came to life, Roxanne began to bleed in spurts from her vagina. At first, we thought she was delivering the placenta. But the placenta had not yet been expelled. So as I worked with the baby, Paula took the necessary steps to stabilize Roxanne, to stop the bleeding, to keep a calm atmosphere around her bed and in the entire room.

Roxanne's mother began to vomit in one corner of the room. The color of her face was a pale ashen hue. Someone quickly gave her a receptacle to complete the task with whatever semblance of dignity could be brought to the rescue.

The New Year's baby was brought into the

world with wide ranging drama. She gave us all a good deal to ponder and reflect upon. As her spirit breathed life into her flaccid body, I saw beyond doubt the meaning of a new life, a new year, a new day.

Every moment is an experience of Eternal Life.

How To Connect With Kate:

http://katelovingshenk.com Subscribe and receive a free report called: 22 KEYS TO SELF HEALING, plus Prayer Prescriptions Delivered to you by email nearly every day!

http://katelovingshenk.com/contact

Facebook Fan Pages: Kate's Radio Show Fan Page

https://www.facebook.com/KateLovingCreativeWisdom

Kate's Author Page: https://www.facebook.com/kate2233

Kate's Blue Heron Farm Spiritual Retreat Center Fan Page On Facebook:

https://www.facebook.com/BlueHeronFarmRetreat

Kate's Prayer Prescription For Nurse Healer Fan Page On Face Book: https://www.facebook.com/PrayerPrescriptionsForNurseHealers?ref=hl

Twitter: https://twitter.com/kateloving

Linked In:

http://www.linkedin.com/in/katelovingshenk22

PRAYER PRESCRIPTIONS FOR NURSE HEALERS is the first in a series. The next book is called: *PRAYER PRESCRIPTIONS: SPIRITUAL REMEDIES FOR LONG LASTING HEALTH.* I plan to write *PRAYER PRESCRIPTIONS FOR AGING GRACEFULLY , PRAYER PRESCRIPTIONS FOR THE LOVE OF OUR ANIMAL COMPANIONS , PRAYER PRESCRIPTIONS FOR VAGINA SISTERHOOD, A MANIFESTO FOR NURSES*

Bibliography

Books That Shaped My Thinking For This Book

Bartholomew, Kathleen
ENDING NURSE-TO-NURSE HOSTILITY: WHY NURSES EAT THEIR YOUNG AND EACH OTHER
HCPro Inc,, 2006

Csikszentmihalyl, Mihaly
Flow: The Psychology Of Optimal Experience
Harper Perennial Modern Classics, 2008

Dass, Ram
Remember, Be Here Now
Hanuman Foundation, 1971

--*How Can I Help? Stories And Reflections On Service*
Knopf, 1985

Laskow, Leonard
Healing With Love: A Break Through Mind/Body Medical Program For Healing Yourself And Others
Authors Choice Press, 2007

Wise, Steven M.
Rattling The Cage: Toward Legal Rights For Animals San Val, 2001

Yogananda, Paramahansa
Autobiography Of A Yogi
Crystal Clarity Publishers, 2005

www.ingramcontent.com/pod-product-compliance
Lightning Source LLC
Chambersburg PA
CBHW061507180526
45171CB00001B/77